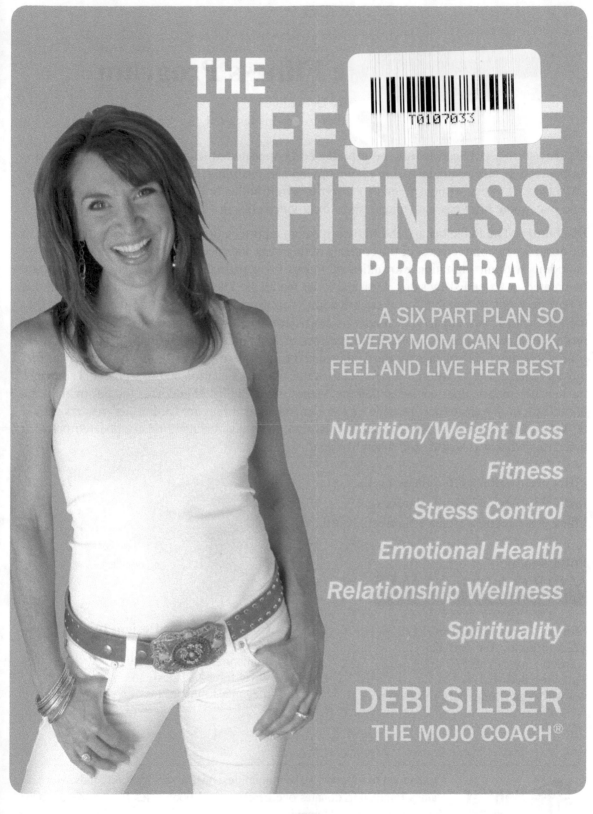

THE LIFESTYLE FITNESS PROGRAM

PROGRAM

A SIX PART PLAN SO EVERY MOM CAN LOOK, FEEL AND LIVE HER BEST

Nutrition/Weight Loss

Fitness

Stress Control

Emotional Health

Relationship Wellness

Spirituality

DEBI SILBER
THE MOJO COACH®

New York

The Lifestyle Fitness Program

By Debi Silber

ISBN 978-1-60037-426-5 (Paperback)
ISBN 978-1-60037-427-2 (Hardcover)
Library of Congress Control Number: 2008923017

Published by:

MORGAN · JAMES
THE ENTREPRENEURIAL PUBLISHER ™
www.morganjamespublishing.com

Morgan James Publishing, LLC
1225 Franklin Ave. Ste 325
Garden City, NY 11530-1693
Toll Free 800-485-4943
www.MorganJamesPublishing.com

Cover & Interior Designs by:
Megan Johnson
Johnson2Design
www.Johnson2Design.com
megan@Johnson2Design.com

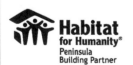
Habitat
for Humanity®
Peninsula
Building Partner

In an effort to support local communities, raise awareness and funds, Morgan James Publishing donates one percent of all book sales for the life of each book to Habitat for Humanity.

Get involved today, visit **www.HelpHabitatForHumanity.org.**

This book is dedicated in loving memory to my mom, Claire Reisner, who taught me how be a strong, empowered woman by being one herself.

This book is also dedicated to my family: Adam, Dani, Dylan, Camryn and Cole. No words can express how blessed I feel to have all of you in my life.

This book is finally dedicated to each and every mom who struggles to find the right balance between motherhood and womanhood. If I can inspire just one of you realize how beautiful, perfect, and capable you are, this book has served its purpose.

Acknowledgements

This book is a labor of love. For nearly twenty years, I've worked exclusively with moms to inspire and empower them to feel, look, and live their best. While each mom I'd known was so unique, her obstacles all seemed to fall within one of six categories. These categories gave birth to The Lifestyle Fitness Program. By working through these categories slowly and steadily, each mom began "getting her mojo back," which gave birth to a title I lovingly embrace—"The Mojo Coach."

The evolution of this exciting process could never have occurred without the love and support from my husband and best friend Adam. Your unwavering belief in me has encouraged me to be who I am today. I wouldn't want to take this fascinating journey with anyone else by my side. Thanks also to my four precious, "highly spirited" children. Each one of you has such a special place in my heart. Dani Max (DanDan)—you are strong, smart, savvy, and perceptive. You always seem to "get it," and I can't wait to see what you do with the endless possibilities that lay before you. Dylan Jay (Sparky)—your easy, fun, magnetic style is a gift for anyone you meet. It's so easy to see why everyone loves being around you. Camryn Leigh (Sunshine)—when the sun shines after days of rain, everyone feels warm and embraced. That's the feeling you give to others. Cole Logan (Spanky)—your impish ways and devilish charm keep me on my toes. Thanks for being you while providing me with some incredible tales of motherhood. Without my children, I would never have believed the depth of love a mom could feel. Thanks for giving me that gift and pointing me on the path to my true life's purpose.

I also want to thank my in-laws, Lenore (FuFu) and Mike Silber. As you celebrate your fiftieth anniversary, know what incredible role models you are. You've taught me the meaning of marriage and commitment through your loving example while encouraging me to grow and evolve under your gentle care. Thanks to my extended family Chris, Susan, Zachary,

Abigail, Lydia, Josh, Russ, Stacey, Jay, Jamie, Hannah, Shayna, Talia, Margo, Jack, Sissy, Bernie, Rita, Anne. I always feel so loved and included. I want to thank my great friends for always putting up with my nutty ideas and hyper-speed style. I'm privileged to have all of you in my life. Thanks to Cynthia for watching the kids when necessary so I could work on this book. Thanks to Bella who always makes me feel so valued. Thanks to Martha for making me laugh, and thanks to Lucie for showing me the meaning of resilience.

Thanks to my clients/friends who placed their trust in me. The risk was in knowing I wouldn't provide a "quick fix," the reward was found in discovering you had what you needed all along.

Special thanks to Dr. Georgianna Donadio, MSc, DC, Ph.D., and the National Institute of Whole Health. You've provided the missing piece of the puzzle in my mission to empower moms to become their best. You've taught me a new way to think, speak, listen, and coach. I'm grateful for your knowledge, support, and belief in me as my passion and purpose developed and emerged right before your eyes.

Thanks to Jeff Wellington Vice President, Publisher *Parenting Magazine*, Dr. Patricia Ross of Peak Proficiency Solutions, Morgan James Publishing, and everyone else who enabled this book to go from thought to finished product. I'm filled with gratitude, love, and appreciation.

Foreword

Recently, I was interviewed by a national health magazine for an article on the growing popularity of health coaching. The journalist asked, "What makes someone a good coach?" and would I identify a list of things readers can look for in a good health coach.

Having spent the last thirty years developing health coaching and health education curriculums, this was a piece of cake. A good health coach was:

- Properly educated, trained, and credentialed
- Had a minimum of three years work experience
- Was knowledgeable in their specialty area
- Enjoys working with their clients
- Exemplifies their coaching

Most health related interviews for print publications, television or radio follow a standard format, which is to ask an expert for a punch list on a selected topic that will satisfy the busy consumer.

After the list was provided, the writer offered the customary, "Thanks for your time. The fact checkers will call." Then, just as we were about to hang up, he asked if I had a second to answer a quick question *he* was curious about. "What do you think makes a *great* coach?"

A discussion that defines a *great coach* would be more in depth and interesting than a discussion about a *good coach*, but that was not the objective of the article. Knowing from too many interviews that my response to his final question would never make it into print, I debated whether or not to start the discussion.

It is difficult, however, to resist an opportunity to talk about a subject one is passionate about, so we spent the next forty-five minutes talking about just that. Ironically, I had just served as Academic Advisor for one of our Whole Health Coaching graduates, Debi Silber, a Registered Dietitian and Personal Trainer from Long Island, New York. Debi Silber personifies what great health coaching is all about.

From my forty years of experience, one of the cardinal rules of *greatness* in the health arena is first you have to do it wrong before you can get it right. To truly master the art, the science, and the philosophy of a given health-focused specialty an individual has to experience the down side of "practicing," where they are in the practice of being "the expert" and allowing the ego to delude them into believing they are a "healer" of others.

The great coach starts off as a credentialed health-related expert. Then, several years after the roller coaster ride of receiving both credit and blame for their client's choices, they discover what healing and the process towards wholeness is all about.

The great coach is born of a confidence rooted in personal struggle and success, anchored in authentic humility and earned through trial and error.

The great coach knows that only the individual can allow healing and wholeness to take place. No matter how great the facilitator, physician, or coach might be, the client allows this process—or doesn't. It is not about the coach being the creator of change but the coach *owning* that change takes place through *information, inspiration* and *personal accountability*.

Since graduating as a Whole Health Coach, Debi has shared that from her training in whole health: "It seems like I traded an anchor for a pair of wings, and it feels so good to fly! I want to bring this gift to my clients and share how they can create radiant health and emotional abundance for themselves and their families."

If you are reading this foreword it is likely that you have been searching for a way to do just that—create radiant health and emotional abundance while raising a family, working, nourishing your marriage, caring for parents and juggling a million other tasks and details.

The great news is that you are about to experience the very best health coaching from the very best health coach I have been privileged to work with.

As my fifteen-year-old daughter likes to say, Debi Silber is *awesome*. Debi has the training, education, work experience, and passion for her work that sets her apart, and she could be a poster model for health and fitness. She is the mother of four happy children, has a healthy marriage, unstoppable energy, and enthusiasm. And that's not even what makes her a great coach!

Debi is a great coach because she has learned both personally and professionally how to *invite you* into your wholeness, not just tell you what to do. She has learned how to *provide you* with information that allows *you* to choose what and how you craft your health, fitness, and wellness. Debi is able to step back, leave her ego at the door, and *deeply listen* to you, hear what you think, what you want and need, and then respectfully and mindfully provide you with tools for success. What an exquisite gift indeed!

I only wish Debi could have been there when I was struggling to raise my three children. Some closing thoughts to ponder: trust the process, trust Debi, and most of all trust yourself. You are magnificently made, and Debi will help you remember that!

Allow me to share with you some words from our Whole Health philosophy: "In our heart there is a longing for the rapture that comes from embracing our authentic *self*, for in each of us lays the seed of potential for that wondrous possibility!"

Health and blessings on your journey,

Dr. Georgianna Donadio

Program Director

National Institute of Whole Health

Boston, MA

January, 2008

Georgianna Donadio, MSc, DC, Ph.D., began her healthcare career over thirty years ago in nursing. Today she is one of only six Nightingale Scholars in the U.S., and an MNA award-winning nurse advocate. Georgianna is a nationally published integrative health expert, clinical nutritionist, and medical educator who maintains a private practice as a licensed healthcare practitioner in the Boston area. In addition, for twenty years she has hosted the critically acclaimed nationally syndicated cable television program, "Woman to Woman,"® which explores spirituality and health issues for women.

Table of Contents

Your Access to Website Support

Your Key to Open The Door to Online Support With Me

I wanted a way for you to stay accountable while giving you access to every benefit you'd have with me through private coaching. If you'd like to take advantage of this opportunity, here's what you can do:

- Visit the contact page of my website at www.TheMojoCoach.com/contact.php
- Scroll down to where it says "Are you interested in" and find in the dropdown menu item "Telling Debi about success from the book"
- Share your success with me in the box you'll see provided
- Click send and your victory will go directly to me!

• • • • •

In addition, I'd like to personally invite you to enjoy a free report, a free year of weekly email tips on Nutrition/Weight Loss, Fitness, Stress Control, Emotional Health, Relationship Wellness and Spirituality PLUS a free subscription to Mojo Moments, my bi-monthly newsletter written exclusively for moms. All free at www.TheMojoCoach.com.

Introduction

First I wanted to thank you for some wonderful things you just did without you even realizing it. The first thing you did was give me an opportunity to work with you. I've helped thousands of moms in the past, and I look forward to helping you become fit and healthy. The second thing you did was give yourself the opportunity to make lasting lifestyle changes through this workbook and through website support with me. This workbook is meant to be interactive, and I encourage you to take full advantage of the unique way to stay accountable with me. I'll be waiting to hear about your successes and will respond to them as quickly as I can.

The third wonderful thing you did by deciding to make lasting lifestyle changes is improve the lives of everyone you touch. It's no secret that when someone feels physically fit and emotionally strong, they feel more comfortable in their own skin. They are more confident, outgoing, and willing to try new things. They are able to get so much more out of life because they are not preoccupied with feelings of discomfort, self-doubt or anxiety. They are often more optimistic because they see firsthand what they are able to achieve. They set a great example while being positive role models for their family. Please understand that I am not saying that weight loss automatically brings happiness. What I am saying is that the positive changes you make by creating new healthy habits gives you a greater sense of control, confidence, and incentive to keep trying. These changes simply feel good physically and emotionally, and we feel proud and happy with the results they bring. Also, everyone knows that when mom is happy, everyone is happy.

The fourth thing you did by purchasing this workbook was help others less fortunate. Please let me explain. When I started Lifestyle Fitness Inc., I made the decision that half of any profits I made from anything I do went to charity. That means that 50 percent of any profit I may receive from your workbook purchase goes directly to those less fortunate. Besides the support, additional information and resources available to you on the website, I will be writing a monthly newsletter to keep you up to date on interesting facts, ideas, and changes in an industry that progresses with lightening speed. The newsletter will also feature a "mom of the month," a mom who has made the most significant changes in her lifestyle (for her). The "M.O.M" will not only be acknowledged and recognized in the newsletter, but will have an additional reward of being able to donate my monthly profits to a charity of her choice.

In the past, you may have read books featuring the latest weight loss plan or exercise program. Perhaps you read books on managing your stress or creating a healthier lifestyle. These books may have been filled with wonderful tips, suggestions and ideas that could have made a significant impact or impression on you. You may have followed the plan for a while and incorporated some of these new changes into your usual routine. If you did, good for you! If you're like most of us however, you had great intentions but slowly fell off track sometime after turning the last page.

You have tried different plans, tips and strategies in the past but ultimately, they haven't worked for you. Maybe you didn't have the support you needed to continue on your journey to greater health. Maybe there was too much information to take in, leaving you feeling overwhelmed or discouraged. Perhaps your stressful, chaotic life got the best of you and your own self-care took a back seat to the immediacy of daily responsibilities and commitments. Maybe because you didn't have to be accountable to anyone when reading the book, you didn't feel as compelled to stick with it. Finally, there's a good chance that you were asked to make drastic changes to your already overextended and overcommitted lifestyle.

I know there were many books or workbooks you could have chosen but something or someone urged you to buy this one. Maybe you liked the cover, maybe you had a "gut feeling" or maybe it just felt right in your hands. Whatever the reason, trust your instincts. You made a great choice, and I'll do my best to deliver. But before we get started, I want to tell you a little bit about myself so you can feel comfortable with who is giving you all this information.

I'm a Registered Dietitian, Certified Personal Trainer and Whole Health Coach. I'm known as The Mojo Coach® because I inspire and empower moms to get their mojo back! These moms have become fit, healthy, and happy through my Lifestyle Fitness Program. The program works because I understand the specific needs of moms today: information, support, and encouragement in manageable, realistic chunks. The success of my practice has motivated me to reach a larger audience where many more moms can receive the benefits of adopting a healthier lifestyle. So, now that you know my professional side, here's a little bit about me personally.

I understand what you go through as a mom because I'm a mom myself. Besides my practice, I have a husband, four children and four dogs. I'm in deep just like you with work, cleaning, cooking, homework, sports, clubs and play dates. I call it "the four *C*'s": *c*ooking, *c*leaning, *c*arpooling, and *c*aring for others. Once we manage to take care of everyone else, we rarely have the time or strength left to care for ourselves. It's a job we do lovingly, but if we're not careful, it is easy to become consumed with the needs of others while our needs fall by the wayside.

Personally and professionally, I have always felt that it is important to practice what I preach, set a good example and serve as a role model for others and my family. That's what's encouraged me to stay on track with my own diet, fitness, and wellness needs since starting my business and family. Let me give you some examples.

You know how difficult it is to find time for fitness once you've had children. Here are some fun tricks I used to get my own workout done. During the colder weather, I put my kids in a playpen filled with toys, coloring books, and crayons safely next to my treadmill. The kids were able to watch their favorite show at the time as long as they were quiet enough so that I could exercise. If they got too noisy, I would change the channel, and they would have to suffer through my favorite morning news show or the decorating channel! The kids quickly learned to keep the noise level to a minimum for their own enjoyment.

During nicer weather, I would put my two older children in a double jogger, put my third toddler in a backpack on my back, and put my infant in an infant carrier strapped to me in front! I had a portable mirror in the jogger pocket so I could see a "rear view" of my toddler daughter over my shoulder enjoying both nature and a ride on her mom's back. I was pushing about one hundred pounds of children, so I didn't have to walk very fast or far to get a great workout. This unusual workout brought us all closer to nature and my kids were "forced" to spend time with me in a unique and special way. Drivers would honk their horns as they passed, giving me the thumbs up, and I quickly became known as "the fit mom who wears all those kids!"

To ensure healthy eating, I took the kids to the supermarket, and we played our favorite game called "what would mom pick." The premise of the game was that I was vacationing in Europe with my husband while their loving, wonderful grandmother was watching them at home. She was too busy to food shop because she was caring for our dogs so they were in charge of the food shopping task. My role was that of a friendly shopper who's job was to give them advice or ideas if they needed, then bag and pay for the groceries. The kids were encouraged to make healthy choices because the better the choices they made, the better the souvenir mom and dad would bring back from their trip. This game taught them responsibility and gave them a jump start to making better choices where it counts the most—before you bring it home!

Being a mom is an exciting, rewarding, hair raising, frustrating, incredible life altering experience. It doesn't matter whether you are your child's birth mom, step mom, foster mom, mom of an adopted child, or primary caregiver. You are pulled in hundreds of directions, have thousands of responsibilities and often lose the battle to find just minutes for yourself. Or you may be like many moms and not even remember who you are besides being your children's mom. Well, it's your journey too. The better you feel, the better you'll be for everyone else. It's time to discover your best self by using each day as an opportunity for growth, development, and fun. To recognize a challenge as something to overcome instead of something to run from, and to see how each success brings you closer to being the woman you truly want to be.

As moms, we take care of so many people and so many things. We are stretched so thin with all of the responsibilities, commitments, demands, and activities we take on. Think about it. From the minute you wake up, your head is racing with thoughts of how you can possibly get everything done on your ever expanding to-do list. The list begins with getting your children up, dressed, fed, and ready to start their day. By the time the bus arrives or you drop your child off at day care, there's a really good chance that you may already be exhausted! Now add food shopping, cleaning, laundry, scheduling appointments, planning birthday parties, paying bills, returning phone calls, school activities, and any other commitment you may have. If you're working outside your home, you have the additional stress and anxiety of meeting deadlines, impressing clients, appearing professional, and performing "at the top of your game." After your daily responsibilities are complete, you need about ten arms and three cars to tackle after school clubs, activities, sports, homework, projects, dinner, meltdowns, baths, and nighttime rituals.

While this seems like a lot of work, now consider the idea that your children may not want to go along with your well choreographed plan. Their idea of how to start their day may be very different from yours leaving you with the added resistance, frustration, and aggravation that occur when a kink in your plan throws off your schedule. Maybe your toddler doesn't like the breakfast you've prepared and decides to "pour" his own juice or cereal leaving you with a huge mess to contend with. Maybe your daughter insists on wearing the same shirt three days in a row and empties her closet to search for what could have been found easily if she only had asked. Maybe your son forgot to remind you that he volunteered *you* to make cupcakes for a school party that afternoon! While each situation may be minimal in the grand scheme of things, when we are pressured, pulled in a thousand directions, sleep deprived, overextended, and running on empty, any alteration to our tightly scheduled plan may wreak havoc.

Now, if you're a single mom, making sure it all goes smoothly largely falls on you. Besides the demands on your day, you may not have the luxury of any additional help to give yourself a break. If you're married, you have different issues to consider. First there's the workload. Many husbands today are more involved than ever, jumping right in when it comes to changing diapers, running errands, cleaning or putting the kids to bed. The responsibilities are shared, and everyone is happy. Maybe however, your husband isn't as involved as you would like or is parenting in a way that is diametrically opposed to yours. While he may mean well, doing things his way may leave you wondering if you may have been better off without his "help" in the first place!

Besides getting things done, hoping everything and everyone is in one piece by the end of the day, there is the idea that you are supposed to make the right decisions about some of the most important aspects of your family's life. Choices regarding the children's schooling, activities, clubs, teams, and social calendar largely fall on us. Then add the amount of computer, TV or time with friends we allow, the rules we instill, and the behaviors we expect. The pressure to make the right decision may cause us great fear and anxiety. We may feel that one mistake in not signing up for a particular baby class, sport, or PTA event will leave our kids and ourselves entirely behind the eight ball. We may look around and see other moms "doing it all" effortlessly and easily while we're barely able to find two matching socks, which leaves us feeling inadequate and incapable. On top of that, add the list we've created of our own expectations of what motherhood should be.

While our list is always enormous, usually it is unrealistic. Somewhere along the line, we've decided that we are supposed to be, do, and act like "super mom." If we work outside the home, we're supposed to do a great job at work and without any sign of fatigue, then put in another full day with your husband and children the minute we walk through the door.

The change from professional woman to mom is supposed to be effortless as we transform ourselves from one person to the next. If we work part-time, we are supposed to manage both our personal and professional lives with ease because supposedly we have the best of both worlds. If we don't have a paying job, we can't understand how we may struggle with the responsibilities of marriage, home and children. Moms have been doing this for years, why is this all so hard and why do we feel so guilty? Here are a few reasons why.

First of all, one of the biggest problems begins with all of these expectations. Who made all of these expectations? Who decided your kids need to be enrolled in every sport, class, and club there is? Whose idea was it that in order for your children to do well in school, *you* need to do all of their projects? When did it become mandatory to fill your children's schedules so fully that no one has a chance to decompress? Chances are it was you. Of course you're only trying to do what's best for your children, there's no question about that. You love your children and want to give them the best of everything. That being said, it's possible that some of the choices you've made don't support *your* values or beliefs. This conflict leaves us feeling that our lives are harried, out of control, and we begin to feel powerless. These feelings also leave us feeling poorly about ourselves and our choices because they conflict with what really matters most to us. In fact, a recent study was conducted to see if moms were happy and satisfied. The study found that over 75 percent of moms studied said they craved simplicity. They wanted simple, well balanced lives as opposed to the lives they were currently trying to keep up with.

It may be time to reevaluate those expectations. Motherhood is hard, and we could sure use a break. Also, wouldn't you rather impress yourself by what you *can* do rather than be disappointed by all that you didn't do? It's not that you're being easy on yourself by lowering your expectations, you're being realistic. What you stand to gain or lose by the choices you make will show you what's guiding your decisions.

Then there's the idea of where these expectations came from. Maybe they came from looking around at other moms, and the more you compare yourself to them the more you find yourself coming up short. As you wonder how they manage to take on so much while always looking great and seeming so happy, you may feel envious, frustrated, and hopeless. How does she manage to get it all in? How can she look so good while raising young kids? Why are her kids always so well mannered and behaved? Questions like these leave us feeling inadequate and uncomfortable. If we don't have a strong resolve along with a healthy dose of confidence in our choices and abilities, we begin to question our decisions, parenting style, and approach to the way we manage our family, our home, and ourselves. We may even feel bitter, jealous, and resentful in our role as mom if we're not careful. So what can we do? If we can be inspired, educated or motivated by another mom then it's great to look at her for ideas. If however, we feel threatened, jealous or resentful, these strong emotions are telling us it's time to look within.

Being a mom is probably the most challenging yet most rewarding job you will ever have. You are shaping the lives of your children and acting as their most significant role model while trying to maintain some sense of self in the process. As you've already learned, that combination is not easy. So let's say you completely disregard your needs to care for your children. You refer to yourself as "Amanda's mom" instead of using your name. You haven't spoken to your husband about anything other than the kids or mutual responsibilities in days. Maybe you don't exercise, eat healthfully or fail to take the time to put yourself together. While you may feel you are being a caring and selfless mom who doesn't have the time to go to the bathroom in peace, have you considered the message your children may be getting? Why is it that they deserve to sit down for a meal and you don't? Why are they able to wear clothes that make them feel good while you just throw something on? Why do you encourage them to laugh and play while they don't see you laughing all that much yourself? Finally, why do you want them to dance, jump and move their bodies while you may be sitting on the couch?

It's always a big shock when you go on an airplane and you are told that in the event of an emergency, put on your own oxygen mask first. As moms, we rarely consider our own needs. If we do, chances are they are only attended to once everyone else is taken care of. That's why it sounds inconceivable to save yourself before saving your children. But think about it. The better you feel, the better you are for everyone in your care. If you are well rested, you have more patience. If you eat healthier, your body looks and feels better and that gives you more confidence. If you exercise, you have more energy and stamina to tackle your day. If you find ways to manage your stress, improve your emotional outlook, and find time for joy, you are better able to enjoy all of the beauty around you. When you take the time for your own self-care, you send a message to your family and yourself that you're worth it, that you like yourself and that mom needs to be happy too. After all, isn't that how you'd want your kids to feel about themselves?

When you grab hold of that idea, you stop second guessing yourself because you trust yourself and your decisions. You learn that it's okay to make mistakes as long as you take responsibility for them. You learn that you can't control everything, so take charge of what you can control (your habits, behaviors, thoughts, feelings, etc.). You learn to redefine perfect and strive to do the best you can because that's *okay*. Feeling good from the inside out requires some self-love, acceptance, and the willingness to try a new way if the old way isn't working. It boils down to not being "super mom" but being an empowered mom, a mom who doesn't judge her parenting by what others are doing, but forms her decisions based on what feels right according to the specific needs of her family. An empowered mom knows that it's okay to be strict, strong, and/or silly depending on the situation. Finally, an empowered mom knows that the most powerful teaching tool is when she uses herself as an example. If you want to teach the kids compassion, be compassionate to others and yourself. If you want to teach them to be confident, then walk the walk and talk the talk. If you want them to be happy, joyful, spiritual, playful, loving, hard working, honest, reliable, trustworthy, and just, show them how by embracing those qualities yourself.

If you're not feeling great yet, you can and you will by giving yourself an opportunity to become empowered through the workbook and additional support with me. The first step was realizing a change was in order and that feeling brought you to action by purchasing the workbook. Instead of staying where you are with your needs unmet, you trusted yourself to find a way to achieve greater health, happiness, and wellness. Be proud of yourself. You're tackling the greatest challenge there is. I It's not easy, but I promise it's worth it. The challenge is doing the best for your family while remaining loving, true, and kind to yourself. So now that you're ready to make some changes, I'll explain the way the workbook and website are designed to work.

How to Use the Workbook and Website Support

Each week I will ask you to make one change from any one category in the Lifestyle Fitness Program. The six programs are Nutritional Fitness, Physical Fitness, Emotional Fitness, Stress Control Fitness, Relationship Fitness and Spiritual Fitness, and they are all important if you want greater health, happiness, and fulfillment. I could have asked you to tackle each step from beginning to end, in the order they are written, but the workbook is designed to be as unique and individual as you are.

The Lifestyle Fitness Program

We all recognize how the same parent can raise such different children with their own distinct personalities, specialties, needs, and desires. We didn't make cookie-cutter children and we are not cookie-cutter moms. We are each unique, with our own set of circumstances, conditioning and specific obstacles to overcome. For example, the reason why one mom carries extra weight may be largely due to a lack of preplanning, while another mom may be eating because she is angry, sad, lonely, tired or bored. One mom may struggle with a poor self-esteem while another mom has been unable to find an effective strategy for stress control.

While each mom is different, so are her needs. That's why *you* will be designing a program based on your most immediate needs first. No one knows *you* better than *you*. As you chip away at obstacles that have prevented you from success in areas of weight loss, fitness or wellness in the past, I will be giving you suggestions, support, and encouragement to get *your* job done. The suggestions you will find are based on the needs and challenges of hundreds of moms I have worked with over the last seventeen years (as well as challenges I've faced). Of course, if I've left out something that has been beneficial to you, please let me know!

Simply choose from the program that appears to be the greatest challenge for you at the time. Once you choose the program (Nutrition for example), choose only one tip, idea, or suggestion that applies to you (such as emotional eating). Please do not choose more than one idea. With so many demands and responsibilities that come with being a mom, the more you take on, the more likely you are to become overwhelmed and give up before achieving lasting results. So, commit to that one specific idea for an entire week while getting any additional support you need. Check off your commitment to the tip by putting a checkmark next to the weekly goal you'll find at the end of the short chapter. That check binds you to that one idea just as your signature binds you to a contract. Once you've incorporated the tip into your routine and tried it enough times so that it has become a part of your routine for the week, let me know! I will do my best to respond to your success as quickly as possible, celebrating your victory, and motivating you to continue.

If by the end of the week you don't feel that you have conquered the issue, choose it again! If you have mastered that challenge, choose a new tip from another program (or the same if that area is especially challenging) and commit to the new challenge while still implementing the changes you made from the week before. Get the support you need, keep working on the tip from week one and week two. The tip from week one is reinforced while the new tip is implemented. Each week builds on the last, until a series of new healthy habits have firmly replaced the old, destructive ones.

When your new tip is firmly placed within your routine, make sure you share your victory with me! You see, while part of me is the Registered Dietitian and Personal Trainer, another part is the coach and motivator. This means I don't just give information. I'm proud of you. I'm rooting for you, and I'm with you during this process, waiting to hear how the best of you is slowly emerging. The other part of me is the caring mom who wants to make sure you're doing okay. So, while I'm here for you cheering you on and motivating you on your wellness journey, I'll tell you the same thing I tell my kids, "I'll try not to hover."

Nutritional Fitness Program

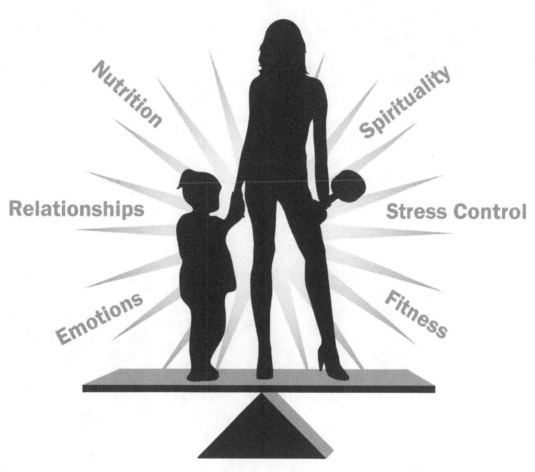

Introduction

I t's not unusual if the mere mention of food sends you running for the hills (or the refrigerator). Most women have an interesting relationship with food. Our relationship began when we were babies. As newborns we had a physical need; our bodies were hungry, and we needed to satisfy that hunger. The physical need was often satisfied along with an emotional need to be loved and cared for. We were given food, and it was served up with love and warmth leaving us feeling nurtured and content.

As we grew, food and love may still have been linked together, and we may have noticed how those around us were affected by this relationship as well. Maybe serving food was a way to show love, eating the food became a way of accepting that love and leaving any over may have meant hurting others by our disregard for their efforts or energy. Besides emotions and food, many of us were taught certain rules and expectations regarding food.

For example, leaving food over was considered wasteful, and we learned to "clean our plates" to please both those around us and the starving kids from a third world country who somehow benefited if we just finished our peas. Dessert may have been used as a reward for eating dinner, finishing a chore or behaving a certain way. We may have learned to "save our appetite" for dinner, eat because the clock says it's lunchtime or eat everything in sight because the "diet starts tomorrow."

Besides certain rules regarding food, many of us could never get enough to eat as food became our closest friend and companion, and we learned to use food as a substitute for what we really needed. We ate when we were sad, lonely, frustrated, angry, bored, or anxious. We looked to food when what we may have needed was a hug, some sleep, a friend, an activity or a better coping strategy. Still others learned to "stuff" their feelings by stuffing themselves.

For this group, the belief was that keeping feelings squelched prevented the pain that may have bubbled to the surface if allowed to express what was building up inside.

Food takes on many roles according to the values, beliefs, habits, and personalities of those around you. If you were raised in a home with few issues regarding food, you may have seen how food still had an important role in daily life, during holidays, celebrations, and special events. Your love for a particular holiday not only involved the people, events, atmosphere, and possibly some gifts, but probably included the special foods and treats associated with it. Food had an important role back then, and it still does now.

Now let's assume you were raised in an environment with food issues ranging from eating disorders such as anorexia or bulimia, restrictive eating, compulsive overeating, binge eating disorder, or any other variation that may exist. Food may have been used as a coping mechanism or used as a way to self-medicate, bringing you immediate feelings of calm, numbness, or relief. Of course the feeling was temporary, and you were left with your original emotion along with shame, disgrace or anger at yourself for choosing such an ineffective strategy. But that's all you knew, and you were just trying to feel better. The way you learned to handle your emotions was something you learned either by those around you, or it was something you taught yourself. In either case, your relationship with food developed over time just like any other relationship. Some relationships are enriching and rewarding while others are dangerous and destructive.

As adults, we're left with the results of the way we've been taught to think, feel, and act around food. Our prior conditioning has either left us with a healthy relationship and regard for food or one that may be completely dysfunctional. In either case, one of the rewards of being an adult is that you have the opportunity to make changes if things in your past no longer suit you. Sure you can blame those who may have shown you some poor eating behaviors but who are you really hurting? By taking responsibility for your eating, giving yourself a little compassion and finding a workable plan you can slowly develop healthier eating habits and behaviors that work *for* you and not *against* you.

For many women, food and emotions are so intertwined it's often difficult to separate one from the other. Through this section, you will learn about *your* relationship with food. You will learn the triggers (people, places, thoughts, and feelings) that trigger you to overeat. You will learn why you choose the foods you do along with the reasons why you eat them. You will become aware of the eating habits you've adopted that cause you to gain weight and lose patience with yourself. You will learn why diets *don't* work. You will learn how when it comes to food, if you fail to plan, you can plan to fail. You will learn how to manage your eating so a binge doesn't derail you. You will learn how to feel satisfied and prevent feeling stuffed. You will learn how to enjoy food in a way that doesn't consume your thoughts, control your actions, and prevent you from living the life you want to live. We have a lot of work to do. Are you ready? Let's get started.

Chapter 1
The Diet Mentality: Deprivation from Food *or* Freedom to Live the Life You Want

Why do you want to lose weight? That may sound like an easy question but I'm looking for more than the "I want to look better" kind of answer. Sure you want to look better but what are your personal reasons for wanting to lose weight? What does looking better offer you? Confidence, improved self-esteem, the ability to be more spontaneous, sexier, more comfortable? Take a minute to dig deep and find *your* motivation to lose weight and the benefits you feel you will gain by losing weight. Go ahead, do it now, I'll wait...

The next question is who are you losing weight for? Some moms want to lose weight for their husband or their kids. Others want to lose weight to impress the neighbors, the tennis pro, women at the gym, their husband's ex-wife and the boy who made fun of them in high school who they'll soon see at the class reunion. It's one thing to have a goal, incentive or motivation to lose weight. Unfortunately however, unless you are losing the weight to please *yourself*, enhance *your* life and improve *your* eating behaviors, your efforts may be short lived. Take another minute to think about who you are losing the weight for.

Now let's talk about dieting. The results are in. Over 95 percent of people who lose weight on diets gain back the weight they've lost plus more in a relatively short amount of time. Weight loss is an over thirty billion dollar a year industry, with plans, pills, and gadgets designed to help us lose weight yet as a nation we're heavier than ever before. The models we see in the magazines are over 5'10" and are a size zero or a size two, yet the average American woman is 5'4" and one-hundred-sixty pounds.

Recent government figures show that over two-thirds of all women are overweight, and 40 percent of girls under ten years old are already on their first diet. Another national survey showed that 94 percent of all moms interviewed claim they don't have enough time to focus on their health, yet 100 percent of those moms felt it was important to set a good example for their families. What kind of example are we setting, and what's going on here?

This is worth repeating, diets don't work. They don't work for many reasons. One of the most important concepts regarding dieting is the concept of deprivation. We think that if we deprive ourselves of the foods we love, we can lose weight. If we deprive ourselves of the social situations where food or drinks are likely to be served, we'll be able to stay on our diet. If our diet food looks, smells, and tastes unlike anything we're used to eating, it's probably good for us and will help us lose weight. If we just have more will power, discipline, and self-control, we'll lose weight. We may be able to follow this path for a while, but I want you to picture something.

Picture a simple rubber band. Every time you are feeling deprived, it's causing the rubber band to stretch. "Can't eat that, it's not on my diet," "I'd love to join you but I may eat something off my diet if I go out to eat," "If it tastes good it's probably not on my diet." Every time you feel deprived, the rubber band stretches and stretches. We may be able to do this for a while, but each time we feel deprived, that rubber band is stretching more and more. The tighter the rubber band is pulled, the more likely it is to snap back. When that rubber band gets pulled as far as it can go, it snaps back with much more force than if it were just tugged on gently. With dieting, we're asking ourselves to make drastic changes and alterations to see results in a short period of time. That's a huge tug on that rubber band. We're expecting (there are those expectations again) results if we simply adhere to the plan whether or not it consists of foods we like or enough calories to fuel our bodies. We may even need to deal with some uncomfortable body issues such as bloating, gas, or bad breath depending on which diet we're on. While we may be able to do this for a while, we eventually give up the diet and go back to our old way of eating (also known as weight cycling or yo-yo dieting). In fact, studies have shown that excessive restriction (dieting) is the most common reason women develop binge eating disorder.

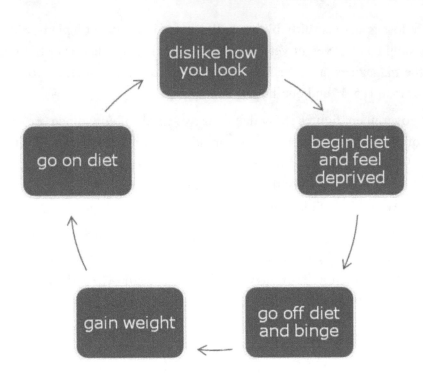

This leaves us feeling as if we've failed; we don't have enough willpower, and we're destined to be overweight and unhappy. Here's the truth. You haven't failed at dieting. It failed you. Diets don't work because dieting means deprivation. As humans, we are naturally pleasure seeking individuals who want to feel good and who don't want to be told what to do. We may deal with restriction for a while, but we'll eventually gravitate towards something that feels more balanced and pleasing. We're also dealing with strong physical, emotional, and psychological triggers that can sabotage our best efforts.

Another reason why the diet failed you is because you were asked to make dramatic changes. Anything drastic is always temporary because it is unpleasant, uncomfortable or just different. We are creatures of habit. Over 90 percent of the way we go through our day is by ritualistic habit. From the way you take your coffee to which shoe you put on first, we barely have to think because it's part of our routine. The foods you prepare, the place you eat, and the manner in which you eat your food are very telling. Good, bad, or otherwise, it's difficult to change so if you're looking to lose weight, the changes have to be gradual enough so that new habits are slowly replacing the old ones.

Diets may also not have worked for you for another reason. Maybe you were able to adhere to a diet requiring severe caloric restriction, excessive food preparation, and extremely limited food choices for a while. But when your day threw you a curve ball—someone or something lead you to fall off track—you wanted to feel better and feel better fast. The diet seemed overwhelming, you wanted relief, and that my friend was the end of your diet.

WEEKLY GOAL

- Do you have a diet mentality? Are you either on or off a diet? This week, remind yourself that diets don't work, and the only way to lose weight successfully is through lifestyle and behavioral change. For now, go back to eating foods you like but commit to leaving two or three bites over at each meal. This tip will slowly break you of having the diet mentality by teaching you that it's okay to eat the foods you enjoy. We'll work on what you're eating another time. For now, lose the diet mentality and enjoy your food—just have less of it.

Another problem that arises from dieting is that we consider certain foods forbidden. These are the foods that we consider decadent and sinful. When we consider foods forbidden, we have instantly given them magical, mystical qualities that are only to be enjoyed once we lose our weight, when no one is looking or as a reward for a hard day. When we eat these foods we may feel guilty, out of control or weak and lacking willpower. This feeling is another sign that we have a "diet mentality." When we do indulge in these foods, we rarely enjoy them because we are busy telling ourselves that we shouldn't be eating it. We haven't given ourselves permission to enjoy it, and we punish ourselves while eating every bite. Sure we ate the food, but we were so wracked with guilt that we never enjoyed it.

WEEKLY GOAL

- There are many ways to make the foods you love taste great while reducing the fat, sugar and calories, and we'll talk about making those changes later on. For now, to help rid yourself of having the "diet mentality" it's important to give yourself permission to indulge in a sweet, delicious, or decadent treat once in a while without any guilt but pure satisfaction so you can get the full benefit it was designed to give. Giving yourself permission to enjoy the treat frees you from feeling restricted while limiting the amount because your decision is one you have planned and allowed for. This week, commit to having a portion size of something you love. Make no excuses, feel no guilt and enjoy it thoroughly. Remember, one portion, one time, and choose something absolutely delicious!

We've talked about the deprivation we feel when we diet, but consider this. If you want to lose weight your eating has to change, that's a given. But while you're making alterations to your diet, making healthier choices, and changing your eating behaviors, instead of looking at what you can't have, how about looking at the confidence, pride, and improved self-esteem you'll feel when new habits are formed? Instead of feeling angry that you can't eat something, how about feeling proud that you're choosing to work towards the body you want? Instead of struggling with the same foods that caused your weight issues for years, how about realizing that these particular foods simply don't work for you, and it's your choice to exclude them from your healthy eating plan? Nothing tastes as good as the feeling of being in control over our choices, our lives and ourselves.

The only real deprivation is not being able to live the life we want due to the pain our relationship with certain foods have caused. Think about how your weight has held you back: relationships, confidence, being more active with your family? Now instead of choosing deprivation, choose freedom to live the life you want by ending the tug of war you feel with certain foods. Not only will it free up some mental space, but it will make you feel like you're the boss, not the chips, cookies, or breadbasket.

WEEKLY GOAL

- Typically, we over-eat the same foods, at the same time, in the same place. Maybe it's the kids snack foods from 3-4PM, the breadbasket on the table on Saturday nights or the late night potato chips we eat while watching TV. Choose which foods simply don't work for you because they are too difficult to control and make the decision to let them go. Sometimes we need to make firm rules with no negotiation. These few foods have held you back from living life the way you want to. Saying no to them means saying yes to freedom! This week, commit to discovering those foods you battle with, recognize they don't work for you, and choose to exclude them from your style of eating.

One of the reasons we may choose a particular diet is because of the structure it offers. For many of us, a structured program gives us guidance and a greater sense of control. Others may find it restrictive and confining, but for those of us who feel comfortable with structure, a plan with set meals and snacks is the way to go.

If you are eating according to your hunger (not appetite, which we'll discuss), you probably find yourself hungry every three to four hours. That means you've fed your body appropriately, it used the calories and nutrients that you've supplied, and it's time for more to ensure your body can keep running and fueling itself properly. If you find that you need more structure, this weekly goal is for you.

WEEKLY GOAL

■ This week, commit to eating three meals and two snacks each day. Control the portions with the meals so you're hungry three to four hours later while making snacks substantial enough to hold you for a few hours as well. We'll talk about food choices later on. For now, commit to eating every few hours while taking notice of your hunger patterns. Were you hungry for the meal or snack? Did you overeat, under eat? Get to know your hunger patterns while nourishing yourself evenly throughout the day.

Let's talk about food diaries. A food diary can give you a much greater understanding of the type and amount of foods you eat. They can track your hunger, your habits, your choices, and your challenges. For many, keeping a food diary is a necessary tool to controlling unplanned or unwanted intake. Many moms have found keeping and recording their food and behaviors crucial to weight loss success. Here's what I've found.

While the food diary tool works wonders for some, it feels very "diet like" to others. It causes many people to become overly focused on the food they eat and the portions they allow themselves. For many moms, the idea of a food diary causes immediate apprehension, resistance, and feelings of failure if they are unable to record their foods accurately and consistently. For these moms, keeping a food diary doesn't encourage lifestyle change because it is yet another unpleasant demand required of them.

WEEKLY GOAL

■ This week, decide if keeping a food diary would help or hurt your weight loss efforts. Sure, it may be difficult to add something else to your list but if this gives you greater awareness and understanding about your habits and yourself, it may be a good idea for *you*. If it is something you can easily incorporate in your day, simply record the foods you are eating while noting if you were hungry for the meal or snack. Use simple codes like H=hungry, N=not hungry, B=bored, A=anxious, D=difficult situation for you (party, eating out, etc.). Commit to keeping a food diary this week if it seems like a helpful tool for *you*.

Chapter 2
Your Diet Legacy and Your Daughter

Since we just finished talking about diets, why they don't work and why they actually cause you to gain weight, I want to give you just one more reason why you need to get off the diet rollercoaster…your daughter. Unfortunately, when it comes to eating, our daughters look to us to see what to do. Now, although our sons are also watching, it seems that as moms, we often pass along our "diet legacy" to our girls almost like it's a natural part of womanhood. Many moms unknowingly teach their daughters that when ready, they'll learn to diet just like their mom.

First of all, I want to start by saying there is no doubt that you mean well. If you were overweight as a child, or are overweight as an adult, you want to spare your daughter the pain you experienced, whether it showed itself through larger clothes, a limited social life, or a low self-esteem. So in order to spare your daughter, you may restrict her choices, monitor her portions, ensure that no unhealthy snack foods enter your home, or just act like the "food police" in general. You may be thinking at this point "I thought I'm *supposed* to only have healthy foods in the house" or "Who else is going to monitor her if I don't?" I'll tell you who—she will.

You see, the more we restrict and control our daughter's behaviors, the less she learns to respect her own internal cues. We all come "wired" to know when we're hungry and when we're full. Think of a baby. They'll cry when they want to eat, and even though there may be only one spoonful left, if they're not hungry anymore they just won't eat it. Their internal cues work perfectly. These cues get thrown off however when we assume control over our daughter's diet.

Just as I explained how the diet mentality is based on restriction and deprivation leading to overeating and bingeing, restricting your daughter works the same way. Time and time again I've worked with well meaning moms who've gone out of their way to "help" their daughters learn to diet. The only outcome I've ever seen is that the more a mom tries to get her daughter to diet, the more it ensures her daughter will be overweight. The same mom who restricts anything with sugar or fat finds candy wrappers in her daughter's backpack, coat or closet. The same mom who limits her daughter's portions finds her overeating whenever she has the opportunity.

Now, I'm certainly not saying to fill your home with truckloads of junk food. What I am saying is that your diet mentality often translates specifically to your daughter. She is on the receiving end of your dieting success or perceived failure. She learns to accept or dislike her body based on your acceptance or disapproval of yours. She will learn to feel bad about indulging in a "forbidden food" if you feel bad about it, and she'll learn that dieting is a natural and expected part of life if it's become a natural and expected part of yours.

The more we diet, especially in front of our daughters, the more we can almost guarantee she'll end up to be a lifelong dieter herself. Girls are dieting at ages younger than ever before. As kids we probably didn't even think about our weight until our teens. Today, girls as young as five or six already "feel fat." These same girls often become confused about what healthy eating is and begin restricting food at an early age. Hungry and unsatisfied from restricting necessary calories, these same girls binge and gain weight. Once they find they're gaining weight they often panic and begin another diet or find something more extreme to help them get the weight off. That's when many girls venture down the dark path of an eating disorder such as anorexia (where there is severe caloric restriction) or bulimia (which involves ingesting huge amounts of food then purging through vomiting or taking laxatives).

No mom wants her daughter inflicted with the pain that a poor self-image can cause. So many factors are out of our control, such as the ultra thin models our girls see in magazines or the skinny celebrity who seems to "have it all." That's why it's important to control what we can...ourselves. Get off the diet rollercoaster if for no other reason than for your daughter. Trust that you're making the right decision by learning to trust your own internal cues and reflect a positive message about the way you think and feel around food.

Find a way to accept your body as it is for now. That doesn't mean you don't want to change it, it just means you don't have to berate yourself for how you look. Remember at all times that you are your daughter's role model. Teach her to not preoccupy her time thinking about food but using food as a delicious form of fuel for her body. You have so many wonderful things to pass along to your daughter, dieting and the pain it causes doesn't have to be one of them.

WEEKLY GOAL

■ This week, commit to resigning from your job as "the food police." Teach by example, not by restriction and control. Your message will get across better and faster if you make healthy, lasting changes yourself. Any change you make must be moderate for it to last. Drastic changes are always temporary. Remember, dieting is not a rite of passage into womanhood, healthy eating and a healthy attitude towards food can be.

Chapter 3
The Food Guide Pyramid: The Basics on Carbohydrates, Protein, and Fat

Y ou probably know which foods belong in what food groups along with what foods contain carbohydrates, protein, sugar, and fat. If you're like many serial dieters, you may even know how many grams of each are in each food! But, for those who need a quick review or summary, here we go.

Carbohydrates fuel our bodies by giving us energy. They come in the form of complex carbohydrates (starches such as wheat in the form of bread, pasta or cereal, rice, barley, and starchy vegetables such as corn or potatoes) or simple carbohydrates (refined sugar, syrup, honey, the sugar found in fruit, molasses, etc.). When carbohydrates are broken down within the body, it is called glucose. Complex carbohydrates are better for us because they contain fiber, which keeps us full longer, and other nutrients that are essential to effectively nourish our bodies. Simple carbohydrates give us that immediate rush but leave us quickly looking for more. The reason is that simple sugars release a surge of insulin within the body. The insulin helps bring glucose to the cells so that cells can get the required fuel they need. When you eat a balanced meal (complex carbohydrates, protein, and fat) adequate insulin is released and glucose can enter the cells. You feel balanced with no sugar highs or lows. With simple carbohydrates, excess insulin is released. Once glucose has entered the cells, the extra insulin will look for something to do. First it will send a message to you telling you to give it more simple carbohydrates. (Ever notice how you have a couple of cookies, then crave some dry cereal, pretzels, crackers or other simple sweets in an often crazed, frenzied way? You're "carbohydrate hopping" and the extra insulin is looking for some carbohydrates to play with). This is a dangerous game because the more you fuel yourself with simple carbohydrates, the more resistant your cells become to accepting what it needs. More and more insulin is released yet not used effectively. Excess glucose is traveling around in the blood which increases our blood sugar level. While extra glucose travels in the blood, cholesterol binds to it easily and makes blood vessels narrower. Over time this can lead to metabolic syndrome (a precursor to diabetes), diabetes, stroke, heart disease and obesity. (We'll talk more about the dangers of simple carbohydrate diets later on).

Next is the protein group. These are either animal or vegetable forms of protein, and they include chicken, fish, beef, pork, eggs, lamb, etc. or vegetable based protein sources such as nuts, seeds, tofu, beans, etc. Protein contains amino acids which repair tissue and aid in growth and development. Protein can be high or low in fat, depending on the type, the cut, the skin and the way it's prepared. Vegetable based proteins are becoming more popular than ever due to the fact that it's relatively inexpensive (a can of beans costs a lot less than a cut of beef) and there are hundreds of ways to prepare them. Great recipes enable tofu to take on almost any flavor while nuts and beans contain important nutrients and compounds.

Protein is a crucial component in any diet. If your body doesn't receive enough protein, it will break down muscle, convert it to glycogen (stored glucose within the muscle) and use it as fuel. Muscle is what fuels your metabolism so less muscle means you require fewer calories. Besides enhancing our shape and tone, we want to preserve muscle to fire up our metabolism while being able to repair muscle and tissues.

Too much protein can be a problem as well. Certain diets require an excess of protein while severely limiting carbohydrates. This type of diet puts an unusual demand on the liver and kidneys by having us lose an excess of water weight which can fool us into thinking we're losing fat. The scale may show pounds lost, but those pounds are largely made up of lost water weight, which is both dangerous and temporary. Water has many important functions within the body, such as controlling heart rate, preventing dehydration, reducing gastrointestinal complications and lessening the severity of skin disorders. If you or a loved one has ever been on a high protein diet, you know there are some very unpleasant side effects of a high protein diet as well.

Another problem with a high protein diet is that it usually discourages the intake of carbohydrates. Carbohydrates fuel your body and your brain. They give us energy, stamina, and they're necessary for a well balanced diet. Eating an excess of protein leaves our diets unhealthy and out of balance.

Now let's talk about the fat group. Fat is an essential part of a healthy diet. It gives many foods their flavor, it's essential for healthy skin and hair and helps us absorb vitamins A, D, E and K, which are known as our fat soluble vitamins. While there are many different types of fat, they each play a role in a healthy diet.

There are two categories of fats. The first category is called unsaturated fats, which are in liquid form at room temperature. Unsaturated fats are either mono or polyunsaturated fats. Monounsaturated fats can be found in olive, canola, and peanut oil, along with avocado and many other nut sources. Monounsaturated fats help lower the bad cholesterol (LDL) while leaving the good cholesterol (HDL) unaffected. Polyunsaturated fats are further broken down into two types, omega-3 and omega-6. Omega-3 fat lowers bad cholesterol while maintaining the level of good cholesterol. It can be found in salmon, tuna, flax seeds, and walnuts. This type of fat helps to reduce tissue inflammation and is important for the health of your cells and immune system. Omega-6 fat helps to lower bad cholesterol, but lowers good cholesterol as well. Safflower, sunflower, and corn oil are popular sources of omega-6 fat.

The other category of fat is called saturated fat, and there are two types, saturated fat and trans fat. Saturated fat is found in fatty meats, full fat milk, yogurt, cheese, and butter. These are your artery clogging fats. They raise bad cholesterol and increase your risk for disease. Trans fat (hydrogenated or partially hydrogenated vegetable oil) is the other type of saturated fat. It is found in certain margarines, fried foods, many packaged baked goods, cookies, and crackers. Trans fat raises bad cholesterol while lowering good cholesterol. Potentially, this may be considered the worst type of fat there is. While we all need fat in our diets, certain fats are found to be more beneficial (unsaturated fats) while others are more harmful (saturated fats). They all can find a place in a healthy diet as long as they are used with consideration and moderation.

A well balanced diet includes foods from all food groups. Complex carbohydrates from the grain group, a variety of deeply colored vegetables from the vegetable group, fresh fruits from the fruit group with a minimal amount of juice, low fat milk sources from the milk group and lean meat, fish, beans, nuts, and seeds from the meat and bean group. While there are many options within each group, it's important to design your diet using foods from each category. For more information on food groups and which foods belong in each group, a helpful website to visit is: www.mypyramid.gov.

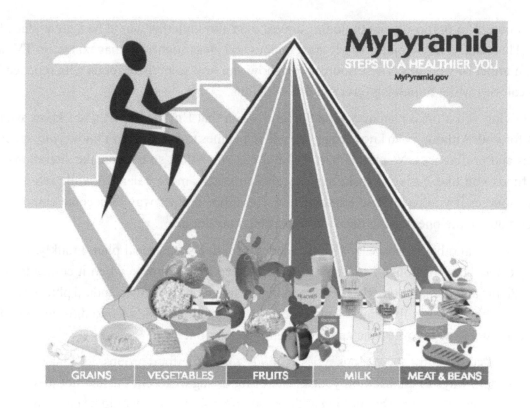

How balanced is your diet? Do your meals contain an adequate amount of carbohydrates, protein and fat? Are you excluding any food group? Are you opting for leaner cuts of meat, lower fat milk sources and plenty of fruits and vegetables? Are you limiting your intake of simple sugar? It's time for a goal.

WEEKLY GOAL

- This week, make sure each meal and snack contains carbohydrates, protein, and some fat. This is usually the most difficult with regards to snacking. For example, instead of an apple, pair it with some low fat cheese. Instead of crackers alone, spread on some peanut butter or have it with a container of low fat yogurt. Commit to meals and snacks that are more balanced. Notice how much more full you feel, how much less you need to feel full, and how you feel more stable, satisfied and balanced.

A note: I'm purposely not including a meal plan although this would be a great place for one. There are so many places to get great recipes and ideas such as in magazines, on TV, and on a number of websites. These sources can show you how to prepare foods with reduced fat and calories while remaining flavorful and delicious.

Giving you a meal plan may give the impression that I'm the expert and I know what's best for you. Although I'm knowledgeable when it comes to food, I don't know *your* specific tastes and preferences. You know best which foods you enjoy, so try to make alterations using foods you like. Strive to make your meals and snacks more balanced while referring to other sources if you're looking for some new ideas. It's another way to become empowered when you are the one making decisions regarding your food.

There is another reason why I've decided not to give you a meal plan. Frankly, I'm not the greatest chef. Although I try, I've learned to keep it real simple when it comes to food ingredients and preparation. My friends and family laugh because my standard phrase is: "I'll cook anything if it has five ingredients or less." It's something that's worked for me, and I'll share a few of my favorite time and ingredient tips later on.

Now that we know the various types of foods within the food groups, let's take a look at some simple ways to cut back on your intake of fat or sugar. To cut the amount of saturated fat, a great place to start is by looking at the meat group. Examples would be choosing leaner cuts of beef such as loin or sirloin, removing skin from chicken and choosing white over dark meat. You can try substituting animal protein with vegetable protein for an additional boost of fiber (beans) and variety (tofu, nuts and meat substitutes).

Another place to cut back on saturated fat is by decreasing the fat content from the milk group. Regular milk can be substituted with lower fat version such as 2 percent, 1 percent skim, or options such as *Skim Plus* that tastes more like fuller fat milk without the fat. Low fat yogurt and cheese options are also available. Be careful with some fat free versions however. While the fat is taken out, sugar is usually put back in. You also may find they are lacking in flavor, texture, or aroma, which may cut calories but may not prove satisfying.

To reduce the sugar in your diet, you want to take a look at the fruit and grain group, along with reviewing the amount of sweets, treats, and extras you may be having. With excess fruit, especially in the form of juice, the calories add up quickly along with the nutrient void refined grains we can easily consume. Review the foods you've been eating for now and here's your weekly goal.

WEEKLY GOAL

- Try to find places in your diet where you can cut the fat and sugar. Maybe you can use light mayonnaise instead of regular, use 1 percent milk in your coffee and enjoy a sugar free frozen yogurt as much as regular ice cream. Find a place to cut the fat and sugar in a way that you can still enjoy the food and not feel like you're on a diet. Commit to one way you will cut the fat and one way you will cut the sugar. That's it, just one way to cut each for now. Commit to the change and don't allow any mental negotiations, deals, allowances, etc. You've made the decision; it's now part of your plan, and it's what you need to do to work towards healthier eating. Feel good about the change.

Chapter 4
Portions and Plate Sizes

Now that you know about the different types of foods, let's talk about portions. First I'll explain what a portion is supposed to be, and then I'll shock you and probably ruin your day by telling you how much we're really eating. Before we begin, I want to explain the difference between a portion and a serving.

A serving is a standard size for an item of food that is published in government documents, on food labels, and typically explained when consulting with a Registered Dietitian. For example, a serving from the grain (carbohydrate) group is one ounce for a slice of bread or one-half cup of cooked rice, cereal or pasta. Serving sizes can be measured by the spoonful (oil), ounces (protein), cup (grains, fruits, vegetables) or by using descriptions such as small, medium or large (whole fruit or vegetable).

We can learn to estimate serving sizes by using familiar objects as measurement tools. For example, one cup is about the size of your fist; three ounces is about the size of a deck of cards, and one tablespoon is about the size of a quarter. We can train ourselves to be more accurate with our measurements by first measuring, then putting the food in a specific plate, cup or bowl. When we see how the serving looks on the plate, cup or bowl we're using, we have a more visual idea of what a serving size actually is. (This is where the shock part usually comes in).

Now let's talk about portions. Portions are not the standard sizes for the foods we eat but are the actual amounts we are consuming. These are the amounts of food we are served at restaurants, eat at home, or indulge in during a holiday meal. When we compare the serving size suggested to the actual portion size we consume, the difference between the two can be staggering.

As a society, we suffer from a terrible case of "portion distortion." While we are super sizing our meals, we are super sizing ourselves. Larger portions are everywhere from the sizes of items offered at the supermarket to the mammoth sized portions we look forward to at our favorite restaurant. I'll give you some terrifying examples.

A medium bagel is supposed to be two ounces. The bagels we eat today weigh in easily at five or six ounces (for many moms, that's almost our grain requirement for the day!). A recommended serving size for pasta is one cup. The average portion size is five cups! A bottle of soda has increased from six and one-half to twenty ounces. A "medium" sized popcorn at the movies now contains sixteen cups and that latte and jumbo muffin you love may cost you more than half of your daily caloric requirements!

Even the sizes of our plates, glasses, and utensils we use have increased dramatically over the years. For example, the average plate size has increased by 36 percent since 1960 with a dinner plate growing from eight to twelve inches. While the sizes of our plates are growing, so are the portions we're eating. (I could have said "so are our bellies, thighs and backsides" but I know you feel bad enough already). Studies have shown that we can eat up to 50 percent more when served larger portions and up to 40 percent more when we reach into large packages or bags ourselves. We're so used to "economy sized" portions, "value meals," and the "bonus" of an extra few ounces on a package, that what was considered normal in the past now looks like a children's meal. So, what can we do?

Our first line of attack is by understanding where portion distortion is affecting you. Is it when you're eating at a restaurant, when you're out, when your home? Once you've discovered where you're overdoing your portions, it's time for a goal.

WEEKLY GOAL

- Although another chapter discusses dining out in detail, we'll mention restaurant portion distortion here. Let's say your meal arrives, and it looks like it's being served on a serving dish you'd use for a holiday meal. Here are a few things you can do. One tip is to avoid having to deal with a huge portion by ordering an appetizer portion instead of an entrée. Another option is asking the waiter or waitress to wrap up half of the meal before it even arrives. Another option is to share an entrée or portion off half and only eat what's left or ask for a salad plate so you can more easily visualize a healthy portion. If restaurant dining provides a portion problem, commit to one of these tips this week. Choose the tip that feels the most comfortable and stick with it.

Let's say your biggest challenge when controlling portions is when you're eating at home. (I'm not talking about binge eating or emotional eating here; we'll get to that later). Here are a few things you may want to try. First of all, check the size of the plates, bowls, cups, and utensils you're using and try to scale down. For example, instead of eating on a dinner plate, use a salad plate that holds less food. Visually, we want to see a full plate. A moderate amount on a large plate can look bigger on a small plate so this trick often works. Another way to design a fuller looking plate is by filling it with a majority of lower calorie items. For example, a high volume of vegetables may have the same number of calories as a small portion of protein. By filling your plate with the lower calorie option, your plate looks plentiful and more visually appealing. Another trick is to use tall, thin glasses instead of short, squatty glasses. This gives the appearance of more while the amount may be the same. Yet another trick is to use a teaspoon instead of a tablespoon and a salad fork instead of a dinner fork. These utensils hold less so they require more effort to eat the same amount. They also encourage you to eat less because taking in the same amount now takes longer. While it takes twenty minutes for your brain to register fullness, smaller utensils take more time to get the job done. (I encouraged a few of my clients to eat their dinners using chopsticks. They learned a new skill while consuming much less than if they were using traditional forks!).

WEEKLY GOAL

- If you find you are using larger plates, bowls, or cups, and eating with larger utensils, start by scaling back. When you're home, commit to using smaller sizes to hold your food and stick to it. If you change from using a dinner plate to a salad plate, commit to the change and stick to it whenever you're home.

This one change alone can save an enormous amount of calories while teaching you what a healthy portion size really looks like.

For many moms, we can gain a greater sense of portion control when we are served less or eat on smaller plates. But what about when we're the one's who are serving the food or when it comes to snacking? Here are a few tips that may help.

Family style eating encourages a warm, friendly, festive atmosphere. Everyone can help themselves and no one has to leave the table. The problem is however, it encourages seconds. When the serving bowls are on the table it's just too easy to reach for more. The food is already there, you're not ready to leave the table and it's easy to overeat. Many moms encourage family style eating as a way to keep the family together at the dinner table. The idea is to be together, not to overeat so you may want to try putting the meal on the plates before bringing them to the table. Everyone can still spend time together without overeating.

WEEKLY GOAL

- If you eat family style at home, this goal is for you. Commit to preparing each plate, and then bring it to the table. The table can still look festive and inviting by using pretty place settings, glasses, etc. The goal is to avoid encouraging seconds from having the food right on the table. This week, no food on the table. Encourage heaping servings of conversation, not food.

Picture a typical meal with your family. (Not the food throwing, screaming, tantrum kind of meal but one that's fairly peaceful and relaxed). Now think about what happens when the meal is over. Some moms encourage their children to clear the table while they clean up and put things away. Many moms however become the human garbage disposal. Maybe your child left over the crust from a grilled cheese sandwich, a chicken nugget, or a few French Fries. Maybe his macaroni and cheese looks delicious or she wouldn't notice if you quickly grabbed a few of her Goldfish crackers. While it may be a bite of this or a taste of that, the calories add up quickly. The best way to see how this looks is by catching another mom eating off of their kid's plates. How does it look when you can look at it objectively? Ugh! If you eat off of your children's, husband's or friend's plates, this goal is for you.

■ First you need to realize that it looks better in the garbage than on you. Next you need to make the decision that if you truly want that food, give yourself a small portion of it and leave your kid's food alone. This week, commit to not touching anyone's food but your own. You can even use the mantra "it looks better in the garbage than on me" if it helps. When there's extra food left over from anyone's plates, have them throw it away if they can, enlist your husband to help, pack, or throw it away before you grab it. Here's where there's no negotiation. No eating off anyone's plates, period.

For many moms, reaching into a bag or a box can be problematic. Serving sizes are small and snack foods are so easy to overeat. What can you do?

One thing you can do is buy portion sizes of the snacks you want. The 100 calorie snack packs are great for controlling portions along with many other single serving sized snacks and desserts that are available today. Another trick is to buy a box of snack sized baggies. When you're *not hungry*, portion the snack from the large bag (let's say you like pretzels and sixteen mini pretzels equals one serving). Make little bags of sixteen pretzels then put all of the snack bags into the large bag. When you go to reach for pretzels, you won't grab an unknown amount but a portion sized snack. By the way, this is a fun project to give small kids. It gives them an opportunity to help mom with a small task while teaching them how to count!

■ Have you found yourself reaching into a bag or box only to stop when it was empty? This week, commit to eating only single servings of snacks and desserts. Get rid of large bags or boxes unless they are either pre portioned or you measure out one serving and put the rest away. While you might spend more money on snack sized baggies you'll save on needless extra portions!

Chapter 5
Our Role in Childhood Obesity

I'm going to begin this chapter by sharing some frightening statistics from the *International Journal of Pediatric Obesity*. Childhood obesity is becoming so prevalent that it is the greatest health risk our kids face today. Did you know that by the year 2010, 50 percent of all children will be overweight? Also, this is the first generation where kids may have a lower life expectancy than their parents! We're spending billions of dollars on healthcare and our kids are unhealthier than ever. What's going on here?

One thing that's going on is that one-third of our children's diets consist of nothing but junk food. Snacks, candy, and other prepackaged foods and desserts filled with fat and sugar supply our kids with a large portion of their daily intake. These sub-foods are nutrient void but dense in calories. That means there's very little quality coming from all these calories.

The next thing that's going on is that while we're suffering from "portion distortion," so are our children. They are learning to super-size, purchase "economy size" and "value sized" meals themselves. They are constantly being bombarded with unhealthy food choices and learning that "the bigger the better." Even if the portions aren't enormous, just take a look at some of the choices available to kids today. It's no mistake that high sugar, high fat foods are at eye level to children at the supermarkets. It's designed that way. This way, when you're shopping with your kids, they can grab it themselves off the shelves, plead, beg and promise until you break down. But where are they learning about all these "foods?"

It's also no mistake that ads for high sugar and high fat food for kids air during your children's favorite TV shows. Just watch some of these commercials. They're filled with bright colors, music, action, and the promise of something special and delicious. They appeal directly to your kids and it's a system that's proved profitable for food companies so it's not likely to stop anytime soon. This brings me to my next point about why more and more children are becoming overweight (hint: it's all that TV).

Think back to when you were a kid. Chances are you played outside with the neighborhood kids after school until it became dark. At that point, all the kids went back to their houses for dinner and you saw them the next day. Today, our kids come home from school and many sit for hours in front of a TV or computer screen. So here's an equation for you. Take a sedentary lifestyle: add a high sugar, high fat sub-food diet to it and what do you get? Overweight kids.

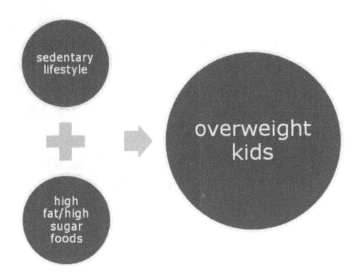

Here's what's also going on. While many kids are sedentary, other children have no downtime at all. They're being shuffled from one activity to the next day in and day out. Now, if you have more than one child that means more shuffling. What are they eating during all of this "shuffle time?" For many moms, the easiest solution is either grabbing fast food to eat on the run or grabbing some snacks for the kids to eat in the car. See where I'm going here?

In our well meaning attempts to give the best to our children, the only way it often becomes humanly possible is by cutting corners. The corners that are often cut show themselves in the food choices we make (for ourselves and our kids) when our lives become hectic and out of control. I'll give you an example of a vivid and embarrassing memory.

Before I understood the importance of a sane lifestyle, downtime and reduced stress, I had my kids enrolled in anything I could sign up for. That meant that from the minute they finished school to the minute they were all sleeping, every minute was accounted for. We either had to be at a game, practice, club, or event often doing homework in the car on the way. Very often I'd have at least one child crying because they just wanted to be home and play. It was timed so perfectly that the minute we would be finished with our last event, I'd rush home and quickly heat up the dinner I'd prepared earlier in the day. I had them wash up, set the table, anything I could keep them busy with during the time I needed to heat up dinner.

One day, I guiltily grabbed some chicken nuggets to "feed" them during our shuffling. As we drove from one activity to the next, I actually started flinging chicken nuggets over my shoulder to my kids in the middle and back rows of my SUV. My heart was pounding because we were running late; the kids were crying because they were tired of all the running around and my aim was so bad that no one could "catch" their dinner! When I had a chance to think about it, I cringed at my actions and behavior. That was my daughter's last day of soccer practice. She doesn't miss it and we haven't looked back since.

My point throughout this chapter is that we all get caught up in "extreme parenting" from time to time. We want what's best for our kids and often sacrifice our sanity, health and well being to give it to them. Unfortunately, our kids may be sacrificing these same things. With this in mind, consider giving them the gift of your positive influence when it comes to their eating, their choices, and their lifestyle. Just know that as you learn about moderation and making healthful changes, your kids can learn too.

WEEKLY GOAL

- This week, commit to identifying how your lifestyle affects your kids and see if it's contributing to the development of unhealthy habits. See what needs to be "tweaked" in order to serve everyone best. It's all about the decisions we make. Just as gradual changes ensure success, this same principle applies to our kids. Moderation is the key and changing poor dietary and sedentary habits now will help spare their health later on.

Chapter 6
Mindful Eating:
Distractions Equal Disaster

When we eat mindfully, many things occur. First of all, we are aware of how much we are eating. We are more in tune with our body signals that tell us when to eat, how much to eat and when our bodies have had enough. We overeat less often because we are paying closer attention to what our bodies need. When we eat mindfully, we are also able to more fully enjoy our food because we are focused on the flavor, texture, aroma, presentation, and atmosphere that surround us and the food we're eating. When we eat mindfully, our bodies are determining when to eat as opposed to the event, the clock, or the show on TV.

Picture a beautifully set table with candles, china and sparkling silverware. Music is playing softly in the background, you're wearing something flattering, your partner tells you how great you look, it was an easy day with the kids, the food looks delicious, you're hungry for your dinner, and you casually stroll to the table for your exquisitely prepared meal. Sounds like it's not that difficult to eat mindfully in this type of scenario, right?

Now back to reality. You're running late and grab something to go, the kids are screaming, the dog is barking, the phone is ringing, and the kids are starving *now!* Maybe you're able to catch a quick break and grab a bag of something crunchy while you read the newspaper. Maybe your hectic day is behind you and you can't think of doing anything else but staring at the TV with a bowl of ice cream in your lap.

To eat mindfully, awareness comes first. You first need to catch yourself eating when you're not hungry. So often we eat mindlessly when we're passing food to others, making snacks for the kids, preparing dinner, walking past the candy dish at work, reading, or watching TV. We may even find ourselves looking to eat when we have a few minutes to spare before our next activity and use food as a way to kill some extra time. Sometimes we may wander into the kitchen, open up the cabinets and wonder why we're even there! I'm not talking about emotional eating where food is used as a coping mechanism offering quick relief or a way to help control your emotional pain. We'll get to that later. I'm talking about mindless eating where distractions and a lack of awareness cause you to take in food when you're not hungry. What can you do?

With greater awareness, you learn more about what you need. When you've learned what your specific needs are, you can work towards solutions that satisfy those needs. So if you're mindlessly eating throughout your day, here are a few ideas to help you become a more conscious eater.

First, stop and ask yourself why you're eating. Believe it or not, you may not even realize you had anything in your hand or your mouth. Ask yourself if you could possibly be thirsty instead. (Our thirst mechanism doesn't always work effectively. We often think we're hungry when we are in fact, thirsty). Next, ask yourself what you really need. If you're bored, you need something to do. If you don't know what you're feeling, you need to figure that out too.

If you're eating just because the food is there, here are a few tricks that have worked for other moms as well as tricks I've used myself. One trick is to chew gum. If you just want to keep your mouth busy, gum may satisfy that oral need. You may also want to use the opportunity to whiten your teeth and put on a strip of tooth whitener. (You can't eat for thirty minutes when they're on). You may find it helpful to keep your hands busy as well. Find things that make it difficult to use your hands by putting on a coat of nail polish, rubbing creamy scented lotion on your hands, knitting, or even wearing rubber kitchen gloves! One client of mine even put on that bad tasting nail polish designed to help you stop biting your nails. It was a quick reminder to not eat and her nails became long and beautiful!

Another trick is to find something to do such as brush the dog's fur, clean a drawer, pop a breath strip on your tongue, or brush your teeth (you may not want to ruin that minty taste). There are also visualizations you can try. Here's one thing you can picture to give you a better idea of how much you're eating. Picture a regular sized plate. Now picture that plate with all of the snacks, bites and treats you grabbed mindlessly. Put on the plate every thing you grabbed when you walked by the candy dish, ate standing up, when you were preparing dinner, talking (and chewing) on the phone, feeding the kids, or watching TV. How does the plate look, is it overflowing?

WEEKLY GOAL

- If you can relate to any of this, use one of these strategies or come up with an effective strategy of your own. The key is to come up with a strategy now so when you need it, it's available. This week, commit to using the strategy you've designed to prevent you from eating mindlessly. Make sure it's something realistic and easy to do. Have what you need available and prepare yourself against mindless munching. If you haven't done it yet, now's a great time to sign up for my free report "Ten Tips To Avoid Weight Gain From Mindless Munching" at www.TheMojoCoach.com.

When learning to eat mindfully, it's important to focus on your food as you eat it. The best way is when you eat slowly, sit down and concentrate on the taste of what you're eating. For many moms however, sitting down to a meal may be a rare treat. By sitting down to a meal, many things happen. First you're becoming more aware of the amount, type, and reasons why you're eating. The second outcome of mindful eating is better digestion. Your food has an opportunity to be chewed, absorbed, and digested more fully. We get more benefit from the nutrients we're eating. Lastly, by eating mindfully you are sending an important message to yourself that you are worthy and deserving of some much needed self-care. You are treating yourself with some kindness and respect which overflows to all those around you.

WEEKLY GOAL

- For those moms who stand when eating, this goal is for you. This week, commit to eating ALL meals and snacks sitting down! It may sound simple but chances are, the standing up and eating habit is deeply ingrained. It doesn't matter if it's even one bite of something, every morsel of food can only be eaten while sitting down. No tasting while you're cooking, no grabbing just one handful as you pass by, no munching as you're making your kids a snack, no excuses period! Every bite, sitting down.

Chapter 7
Out of Sight, Out of Mind

When we are trying to lose weight, people, places, situations and events can sabotage our best efforts. More often however, we sabotage ourselves by making things more difficult than they need to be. When creating new, healthy habits one of the primary goals is to make things easy so your efforts have a payoff and you see results. I'll give you some examples.

Do you notice how you tend to grab more food or snacks just because it's sitting on the counter? How about when you wrap up delicious leftovers from a holiday or party and you know exactly where to find them when the craving calls? Here are a few easy tips to make the food a little less accessible.

First, never leave food out on your counter, table, or desk while at work. It's an open invitation to indulge whenever you glance at it or pass by. The next tip is to wrap foods in aluminum foil instead of saran wrap. By wrapping in aluminum foil, you don't see the food and you are less likely to be affected by it. Another trick I've used is to put tempting food in the refrigerator in my garage (use this tip if you have another refrigerator or storage area). I have a real sweet tooth and I love to bake. Sometimes I purposely bake things I don't like so I'm not tempted by them. If it's something I love, however, I'll store it in the other refrigerator so it's not as accessible. As I walk to the garage, it gives me an opportunity to think about how much I really want it. I can't tell you how many times I've changed my mind on the way to find my hidden treat. The few seconds required to walk into the garage allow you enough time to reconsider. You can also ask your husband or your kids to put the food away and not tell you where it is (my son loves to do this with anything BUT food by hiding my keys, wallet, cell phone, etc.).

WEEKLY GOAL

- This week, commit to putting all food out of harms way. Nothing should be left on countertops, tables, or within easy access. See how much easier it is and how much less you struggle when you are less tempted. When you reach for food it will be more intentional, you've planned and allowed for it. You'll also see that if you're struggling to find and recover hidden food like a crazy person, something deeper may be going on.

Chapter 8
Ride the Crave Wave

What is a craving? According to the dictionary a craving is a desire, wish, hankering, need, or requirement. It's something you lust after, pant, or pine for. These feelings can be so strong, the pull so severe, that we don't feel we have a choice but to give in to whatever the craving is calling for. Now, there's a difference between needing something and wanting something. Your body *needs* food and water in appropriate amounts at regularly scheduled intervals. What your body doesn't need is that triple chocolate cake or that third glass of wine. These feelings can be confusing. Hunger is a physical need. It is your body's way of letting you know that it needs to be fed and it signals you with stomach growling, weakness, and other messages to eat. Appetite however is something different. That's when the desire to eat is in response to something you see, smell, hear, or think about. "Mom, I *need* that new toy!" In this case, understanding the difference between wanting something and needing something becomes crystal clear. So why do we find it so confusing and what can we do?

The first thing you need to do is recognize if the craving is telling you something important. If your stomach is rumbling, you're starting to feel dizzy or light headed, you need food and you must respond to the message your body is sending. If you sense that it is not a physical craving, there is a different approach you can take. For one, you may feel you have no choice when a craving comes on; but you do. You don't have to give in to the craving.

Sometimes drinking water will help. Sometimes distancing or distracting yourself from the food that's calling you can do the trick. Remember when you had contractions when you were in labor? They started out strong, got more intense, peaked, and then slowly reduced in intensity? Cravings work the same way. They come on strong, get even more intense, and then often go away if we become distracted. This may also be a good time to question the craving to see if the real need to satisfy is an emotional one or is in fact a physical one.

Another strategy you can try is having only a taste of whatever it is that you're craving. For some this may be extremely difficult but for others it's the way to go. Denying yourself only increases the intensity of the craving for some, and by having just a little bit, you stop obsessing about the food and satisfy the craving. Sometimes when you give in to these types of cravings and have just a taste, you find that the forbidden food doesn't taste nearly as good as you'd imagined! If you can satisfy your craving by having a taste, here's an important concept to remember as well.

The idea is to satisfy the taste so it's over with, out of your head, and you can focus on something else. One or two bites should do the trick if you eat them slowly and mindfully. Remember however that the third, fourth, and fifth bite tastes the same as the first but by having more than a few bites you might start paying the price by wearing it on your thighs. If you can satisfy the craving with a bite or two, give into the craving and then let it go.

Finally, you may crave things that are extremely sweet, salty or creamy. This is often a sign of a craving driven by emotions. Studies have shown that certain tastes and textures are indicative of certain emotions. For example, people choose salty, crunchy foods when they're stressed or angry, while others choose sugary, creamy foods when they're lonely or depressed. Like everything we've discussed so far, the key is to become aware of how you're thinking, feeling and acting so you can devise the most effective game plan for you. If you battle with cravings, this goal is for *you*.

WEEKLY GOAL

- This week, recognize what's going on when a craving hits. Did you wait too long between meals? Is there a pattern as to what you're craving and when you're experiencing cravings? Identify if it's a physical need for food, if the desire was a response to something you've heard, smelled, or seen, or if it's an emotional craving. If it's physical, respond to the need. If it's emotional, try to identify what it is that you really need. If it's just something that you want, ride the crave wave or satisfy the craving by having a small amount. Commit to identifying your cravings and riding the "I just want it" kind by using distraction techniques or distancing yourself from the food. If you're able to have just a small amount, satisfy the craving and move on.

Chapter 9
Becoming Supermarket Savvy

One of the easiest ways to avoid temptation is to avoid bringing high fat, high sugar foods into your home in the first place. This effort begins at the supermarket. Studies have shown that moms make over 90 percent of the food purchasing decisions, so learning how to food shop more effectively can be a useful skill when trying to create new, healthy lifestyle habits.

The first step is to avoid the impulse, random purchasing of binge type, trigger foods. The easiest way to do this is by shopping with a prepared list. Lists don't have to be written out at one time. This may be perceived as a big task. An easy trick is to keep a running list easily accessible in your kitchen. When you're running low on something, jot it down. When a meal idea comes to mind, write down the ingredients. When you see a picture, advertisement, or commercial with beautiful fruit, vegetables, or a delicious looking healthy meal grab your list and write down what you'll need to enjoy the same foods you're seeing in the magazines and on TV.

The next step is to take *only* your list to the supermarket. Leave your hunger at home and don't bring the kids if you can help it. When you food shop and you're hungry, you're much more tempted to buy things you would normally bypass if you were satisfied. By having a light snack or mini meal before you enter the supermarket you are able to make more sound choices with your judgment still intact.

Have you ever noticed how much more junk food you buy when you bring your kids to the supermarket with you? "Mom, can you *pleeeeeease* buy this (sugary, calorie laden) cereal I saw on a commercial?" "Mom, everyone brings in these (high fat, high cholesterol, nutrient void) snacks to school!" The battles can be endless in the supermarket, with foods containing the least nutrition and most fat, sugar and calories strategically placed right at your children's eye level. If you must bring your children, bring a strong resolve to stick mostly with your list, but if you have a choice, use the opportunity to make better choices while catching a few moments for yourself.

So you're armed and ready, where do you begin? First let's talk about labels. The first thing to notice when looking at a label is to note the number of servings per item. The calories, fat, cholesterol, fiber and sodium are listed for one serving only. So for example, if you buy a bag of popcorn, the bag contains ten servings and you finish the bag, the calories, fat, cholesterol, and other nutritional information must be multiplied by ten. Also, with regard to labels, ingredients are listed in order of the highest concentration to the least concentration. This means that if sugar or fat is listed within the first few ingredients, there's a high concentration of sugar or fat in the item. Also when you're reading labels, know that sugar is often disguised under many different names. Anything containing high fructose corn syrup, any nutrient ending in "ose," honey, molasses, fruit juice concentrate, and brown sugar are forms of sugar that act just like regular white, refined sugar within your body.

When looking at ingredients on the label, how many look familiar? How many can you pronounce? How many would you feel comfortable adding to something you were cooking or baking at home? When you were a child and your grandmother baked her delicious, mouth watering apple pie, the only flavor enhancer she added was the love that went into baking it for you. Although there are thousands of items available to us today, an alarming amount are pre-packaged, processed, and provide little nutrient value. For example, when a food is processed, it's been altered from its natural state. Valuable nutrients, vitamins and minerals are taken out while chemicals and additives are injected back in. Food dyes, flavor enhancers, stabilizers and preservatives may make food look more colorful or extend shelf life but think about it. If a product can last indefinitely on a store, vending machine, gas station, or food court shelf, what happens to it when it's within your body? An easy rule to make healthier purchasing choices may be this: if you can't pronounce it, if you wouldn't add it to anything you were cooking or baking at home, if you wouldn't find the ingredient in your favorite cookbook, it's probably best not to eat it.

So what are the healthiest choices to make when food shopping? Most of the healthiest foods are located on the outermost aisles. These include your fruit, vegetable, dairy and meat departments. Let's start in the produce department.

Here's where you want to really fill up your cart. Fill it with beautiful, interesting and colorful fruits and vegetables. Different colors of fruits and vegetables offer different nutrients so just by making colorful selections, you're automatically increasing your chances of getting a wider variety of healthy nutrients. There are also many varieties of pre-washed, precut lettuces and other vegetables that make it easy to prepare interesting salads and vegetable dishes. Here's where you splurge, because if a variety of pretty, precut vegetables are available at home, you may reconsider eating pre packaged, processed junk food.

In the meat section, opt for leaner cuts of beef, chicken and turkey. Choose cuts with less visible fat to decrease your intake of saturated fat. With fish however, choose both fatty (salmon and tuna) and lean varieties. Fatty fish are great sources of omega 3's and white colored varieties (flounder, sole, and halibut) are low in fat and calories.

In the dairy section, look for words such as low fat, non fat, and fat free, 1 percent, 2 percent, and skim. Eggs, butter, margarine, and soy products are usually in these aisles so read labels and choose carefully. Watch the fat when choosing milk, butter, margarine, sour cream, and cheeses, along with looking out for sugar added to yogurts, creamers, and soy milk.

You can still pick up healthy items in the center aisles if you choose carefully. In the grain aisle, try to avoid refined carbohydrates and opt for whole grain and high fiber whenever possible. Choose 100 whole-wheat bread, high-fiber cereals, whole-grain pasta, brown rice or sprouted-grain bread. The closer the grain is to its most natural source, the more fiber and nutrients it contains. Beans can also be found in either the grain or canned aisles. Dry beans require soaking, which may not appeal to you. Canned beans are just as nutritious, so if you'll eat more beans this way, buy the canned versions. In the frozen section, you may want to grab a few bags of frozen vegetables or mixed blends (without the added sauces or butter flavoring). Frozen vegetables retain the vitamins and nutrients while being convenient and easy to prepare.

When you become more familiar with labels, packaging, and products, you begin to realize that the supermarket can be either a health promoting environment or a war zone where you battle with your best intentions, your cravings, and your judgment. If you can use some supermarket savvy, this goal is for you.

WEEKLY GOAL

- Do you use a shopping list? Are you label conscious? Do you buy the majority of your foods from the inside aisles? This week, use a food shopping list. Stick to the list and only buy extra if it's something nutritious. Look for ingredients in your food that sound like something you'd cook with. Shop mostly on the outer aisles and choose carefully in the center aisles. Try a new fruit or vegetable. The goal is to become more aware of the foods you choose so you're less likely to be blindsided by them once they're within your home. Commit to filling your cart with more fresh produce, healthier snacks and lower fat meats and dairy. This week, commit to filling your cart so you're proud of your choices as you unload them onto the turnstile. If you need some extra help in this area, consider my "supermarket savvy food shopping tour." You'll learn to shop easily and effectively according to your needs, time, budget and lifestyle. Email Info@TheMojoCoach.com for more information.

Chapter 10
Tips For Traveling, Restaurants, Weekends and Parties

For many of us, eating outside the home can prove disastrous. Vacations mean a vacation from healthy eating, and navigating our way through a restaurant menu can seem daunting. Here are a few suggestions to ensure a better outcome the next time you eat away from home.

While vacations offer time off from our daily responsibilities and commitments, they often mean time off from healthy eating as well. If you find vacations give you a great excuse for some "time off" from healthy eating, you may want to consider if your eating style was too restrictive. When you're making lasting lifestyle changes to your diet, there is never a reason to be "on" or "off" because you've allowed for some flexibility and imperfection. Eating dessert isn't a tragedy because you simply understand that you've allowed for it or you'll cut back during the next meal. With healthy lifestyle changes as opposed to dieting, you've also given yourself permission to indulge every so often, which often eliminates the need to binge.

Weekend eating is often similar to eating on vacation because of the lack of structure a weekend often provides. The same ideas apply here. Allow for some imperfection to avoid the need to binge. It's also important to pre plan for overeating whenever you can so you have a strategy when confronted with excess food. For example, let's say you enjoy drinking on Saturday nights and you usually drink more than you'd like. Decide before you head out that you'll have one glass of wine and alternate sips of wine with a glass of water or choose a wine spritzer to cut the amount of wine instead. If you're headed to an affair where buffet tables will be overflowing with delicious treats, there are a few strategies you can try as well.

The first thing you may want to try is to never go to an affair with a roaring appetite. It's too easy to overindulge and by having a small snack, you'll have a clearer perspective and make better choices. Another trick is to have a drink in one hand (you can have a club soda, which looks like a drink, and no one will bother you about not drinking) and carry a clutch purse in the other. Now you have no free hands to overeat! A third trick is to carry the drink or clutch in one hand and fill a plate with vegetables for the other hand. Now you're eating with minimal damage. You can also pre-plan before the event that you will allow yourself to try three incredible looking appetizers or desserts. Taste each one, savor the flavor and enjoy! When it's time to sit down for the meal, leave over what looks ordinary. Use the opportunity to try unusual, interesting foods while avoiding excess calories from foods you already know and have tasted many times before. Now that you have some tips for vacations, weekends and parties, what about when you go to a restaurant?

Here are a few things you can try. In chapter four we covered ideas such as sharing entrees, ordering appetizer portions, etc. While those ideas may come in handy, there are a few words to watch for when ordering. Look for words such as baked, broiled, roasted, grilled, poached, seared, or steamed. While herbs, spices and seasoning are used, these words usually mean the food is prepared with less fat. Words such as sautéed, fried, creamy, battered, or cheesy usually describe a food filled with fat and calories. If you choose these items, watch your portions by making the decision to leave some over, order sauces on the side and compensate for the excess before, during, or after the meal.

To prevent overeating, you may want to start with a clear, broth based soup or a salad. When ordering a salad, asking for dressing on the side is another helpful way to control portions. Order a dressing that you like. Salad is too important to be turned off to by a poor tasting dressing. To limit using excess, order on the side then dip your fork in *first*, before putting the salad on the fork. You'd be amazed at how much less you use while still enjoying the flavor you love. When you want to *stop* eating, you need a game plan as well.

You can put the opposite ends of the utensils on your plate (so they touch your food and they're unpleasant to pick up), pour water, salt or pepper on the dish, cover your plate with a napkin or simply push it away. I had one client who always made a statement like "wow that was great, I'm stuffed" at the end of her meal. Once you've announced that you're finished, you may feel uncomfortable reaching back into your plate. You may also want to keep in mind that most waiters and waitresses have heard special requests before. They can handle it so don't be afraid to ask. While it may feel uncomfortable to ask for things on the side or to have foods prepared a certain way, if you choose not to the only person you're not accommodating is yourself. Here's your goal.

WEEKLY GOAL

- What happens to you on vacation, parties, affairs, restaurants? Take the time to assess how you handle yourself and decide on a solution that keeps you on course whether it's coming up with your own phrase when out, ordering foods on the side, covering the plate, etc. By having your strategy readily available you can use it when the time comes and avoid paying for it later. This week commit to a strategy when dining out, vacationing, parties, weekends or whenever you are tempted to overindulge. Have your strategy firmly in place and use it accordingly.

Chapter 11
Lapse, Relapse and Collapse Behavior

When you look at the weight fluctuations of naturally thin people, their weight typically fluctuates within a few pounds. Maybe they might gain a pound or two over vacation, during a holiday season or even after a weekend of overeating. When they feel their weight may have crept up a bit, they pull back on excessive overeating, over-drinking, and over-partying and gradually find their most comfortable weight.

One of the greatest differences between someone who's naturally thin and someone with excess weight to lose is the point at which they decide it's time to end the overeating and lose the weight. A thin person may begin to feel uncomfortable after gaining three pounds where an overweight person may decide that "enough is enough" after gaining twenty, fifty or one hundred pounds. That point varies from person to person because we all have different comfort levels. The point is, whatever weight gain makes you feel uncomfortable, unhealthy, and unattractive is the place where working towards healthy eating often begins.

Are you an all-or-nothing dieter? Many of us have become so accustomed to dieting that we are always on or off a diet at any given time. This all-or-nothing behavior only sets us up for failure because the expectation is that if we are not perfect, we've blown the diet and all that's left to do is give up. Fluctuations in weight and eating behaviors are normal and are more in line with making lifestyle changes. When you find a middle ground, set reasonable goals and realistic expectations, there is a much greater likelihood of encouraging new behaviors to emerge. Think about it. If you're making better choices and you give in to that delicious dessert (lapse) many of us decide that we may as well go back to eating the foods we've so carefully limited (relapse) and then just give up our efforts altogether (collapse). So instead of dealing with the possibility of a half or one pound weight gain, we may as well gain back the whole amount. Does this make any sense?

The trick to avoid a dietary disaster is to prevent a slip from turning into a fall and then tumbling down the entire mountain. Simply contain the slip to the meal, the event or the situation. Make sure there's a definite conclusion. Don't berate yourself, and get back on track. There isn't one positive outcome that can come from being disgusted with yourself for the lapse, so do your best to let it go. If it helps you, you can also use the three to one rule. Here you compensate three healthy choices for the one unhealthy choice or three healthy meals to compensate for the one meal you'd rather forget. The three to one rule is a useful tool to balance unhealthy choices and bring healthier choices back into place.

WEEKLY GOAL

■ How's your eating style? Is it all-or-nothing or do you allow for some imperfection once in a while? When you fall off track, what do you do? At what point do you stop the slip from turning into a fall? This week, determine your eating behavior when you fall off track. When you slip (we all do), commit to stopping the lapse from turning into a relapse or collapse. Quickly contain the lapse, assess what happened while being compassionate with yourself and get back on track. Learn from the lapse and renew your commitment. A lapse doesn't mean the end of healthy eating. It's just a new starting point for regaining control.

Chapter 12
Breakfast Like a Queen, Lunch Like a Princess, Dinner Like a Pauper

You've probably heard that breakfast is important for weight loss for many reasons. One of the most important reasons to have breakfast is that it ends the body's notion that you're fasting. Overnight, your body perceives a moderate fast so your metabolism is slowly reduced in order to conserve energy. It's a protective mechanism to help prevent your body from starving (how thoughtful)! When you fuel you body with breakfast, your metabolism is fired up and this protective calorie sparing mechanism is put to rest. Breakfast can also be a relatively easy meal to control when it comes to portions, fat, sugar, and overall calories if chosen with care. It's typically also a manageable meal offering you a great place to fuel up on quality protein, high fiber grains, fruit, and low fat dairy.

Many of us however, fail to eat breakfast or believe we'll help ourselves if we simply skip this meal because we may not be hungry for it. Studies have shown that breakfast eaters weigh less than non breakfast eaters. Breakfast eaters also tend to take in more fiber in their diets while eating less fat and calories throughout the day. When you choose to ignore breakfast, your body hasn't ended its fast (break-fast) but by skipping meals your hunger will eventually return—and with a vengeance. Now the choices are more limited, more fattening, more sugary and caloric. Plus, you're starving! When we're hungry, our reasoning, judgment, and best intentions go astray. Our choices are based on what is the most convenient and accessible rather than what is best for us.

Healthy Eating Style

Unhealthy Eating Style

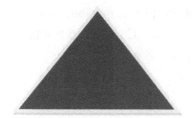

DINNER

LUNCH

BREAKFAST

With regard to choice, another point worth mentioning is our choice of beverages. As a Registered Dietitian, I would always encourage you to eat the fruit instead of drinking its juice. Juice contains concentrated calories while limiting nutritious vitamins, minerals, and compounds found in the fruit skin and within the fruit itself. For example, one 8 ounce glass of orange juice contains the same amount of calories as two oranges. It may be easy to drink a glass of juice but you may not consider eating more than one orange. It's also more satisfying to chew your calories rather than drink them. Many other drinks (soda, blended coffee drinks, shakes) can be caloric time bombs as well. One loaded blended coffee can contain over seven hundred calories! While often delicious, it's important to use discretion when choosing liquid calories.

Studies have also shown that for those who don't eat breakfast, more than 50 percent of total daily calories are consumed towards the end of the day. When you eat earlier in the day, you have more of an opportunity to evenly distribute your calories so you can utilize calories instead of storing them as fat. Your body functions at its best when calories are distributed more evenly throughout the day. Blood sugar levels remain at a constant, energy is burned versus stored and sufficient energy is supplied to encourage organs and body systems to function optimally. Are you eating breakfast like a Queen? Time for a goal.

WEEKLY GOAL

- If you're not a breakfast eater, this goal is for you. One reason you may not want breakfast is that you're not hungry for it. One idea is to stop eating three hours before bedtime to get your body more in line with waking up hungry. Next, you can choose a small serving from the grain group and make sure you balance it with some protein (ex: container of yogurt with fruit, one-half bagel with peanut butter, one piece of toast with low fat cheese). Commit to breaking your nightly fast to ensure a metabolism that's ready to go.

Chapter 13
The Dangerous Side of a High Sugar Diet

Although we previously covered the basics regarding sugar (in the form of simple carbohydrates) it's beneficial to know the physical and emotional consequences of a diet high in refined, processed sugar. Physically, refined carbohydrates promote an excess secretion of insulin which taxes the pancreas. Glucose (sugar within the body) travels freely and becomes unable to enter and nourish cells. When this occurs, obesity, insulin resistance, metabolic syndrome, and diabetes are often the result of this malfunction.

Another physical reaction to an excess of sugar is the secretion of the stress hormone, cortisol. Along with many other functions, cortisol increases appetite and food cravings that lead to weight gain (we'll talk much more about the dangers of over secreting hormones in the stress control section). A further physical complication of a high sugar diet is the onset of hypoglycemic and hyperglycemic reactions caused by the dramatic fluctuations between blood sugar levels. These fluctuations create severe mood and behavioral disturbances, making us feel shaky, lethargic, moody, and unstable. In an effort to feel better, we often reach for nutritionally depleted, high sugar, easily ingestible foods for an instant energy surge. While we receive a quick boost of energy from these foods, it is short lived and we often live from surge to surge on a roller coaster ride of sugar induced energy. This type of diet also stresses the immune system. The immune system acts as the night watchman of the body, protecting it against unwanted invasion. When it becomes taxed or stressed as with a high sugar diet, it is unable to work effectively, causing inflammation (which interferes with the hormones designed to help control appetite and metabolism) creating numerous health related conditions and disease. We spoke about mixing carbohydrates with protein and fat earlier, along with eating every few hours to avoid a possible binge. This weekly goal is for those who experience the highs and lows of a sugar take off and crash.

WEEKLY GOAL

- Do you eat a diet high in refined, processed sugar? Have you ever felt shaky and anxious, feeling the need to eat large amounts of simple carbohydrates quickly? While simple carbohydrates are easily accessible, release the feel-good hormone serotonin and provide instant energy, they leave you to crash and burn. This week, commit to not going longer than three to four hours without a meal, making sure you choose whole grain, higher fiber more complex carbohydrates and eat your carbohydrate choice with quality low fat protein. Commit to more well balanced meals and snacks and note how much more calm and balanced you feel both mentally and physically.

Chapter 14
Emotional Eating

Let's say you are stressed, frustrated, angry, sad, lonely, tired, or depressed. You want to feel better and it's an automatic reaction to reach for foods filled with sugar and fat. This is emotional eating and a few things are happening here. First, you're trying to find a fast, easy way to self-soothe that doesn't require any thought or pre-planning. It's easy; it temporarily numbs the pain, calms the anxiety, reduces the anger, keeps the fear down, and provides a temporary distraction so you don't have to evaluate, fix, or solve your problem. Yes it keeps you overweight, but it also provides an opportunity to remove yourself from feeling, thinking and dealing with your fears, doubts, and insecurities. You may be unaware that you even do this, or you may not know why you've chosen this coping strategy. What you do know is that by taking the path of least resistance with emotional eating you remain overweight and unhappy.

Every reason why we eat emotionally offers valuable clues as to what it is we really need. The least it shows us is the need to pre-plan. More often, emotional eating occurs to fill a void for something we feel is missing from our lives. Whatever the reason, it leaves us feeling empty, uncomfortable and out of control. So what can you do?

First of all, berating yourself for binging only encourages another binge. Remember, it is a self-soothing technique you have employed to help yourself feel better. Imagine a hurt child who's trying to tell you why she's hurt. Typically, telling you her story is the first step to feeling better. Once she feels heard, she feels as if a weight has been lifted. She feels understood, validated, loved and can happily move on after a few minutes of explaining her feelings and receiving a supportive hug from someone who cares. Now imagine that same child but instead of listening to her "crisis," you forbid her from explaining her pain or feeling her emotions, and you choose to feed her instead. How does she feel?

- She's frustrated with the feeling of being squelched.
- She's unlikely to feel better because she's still dealing with emotions that haven't been adequately felt and dealt with.
- She's never had an opportunity to resolve the conflict that caused the pain so the painful feelings remain.
- She feels hopeless that this feeling will ever change.

This is what we do to ourselves when we binge. We squelch that hurt child and fail to uncover the unmet need. The need remains unmet; we remain unhappy, unfulfilled, and overweight. This cycle of binge, feel bad, binge again is a cycle leading to nowhere but bigger clothes and poor self-esteem.

There are a multitude of reasons why we may eat emotionally, ranging from staying with conditioned behaviors we were taught to having insufficient coping skills or outlets to help us handle our problems and ourselves in a more effective way. While it seems natural to want to kick the emotional eating habit in order to lose weight, many of us may need to consider why we may feel the need to keep the weight *on*.

Weight provides a protective barrier. Remember when you used to hide behind your mom's leg when you were scared? Our extra layers of weight may be providing that same security. For many, losing weight may leave us feeling insecure or uncertain because our role may change once the weight is lost. Expectations by others and ourselves may change as a result of weight loss success and we may feel compelled to accomplish more, perform, or behave differently as a result. This feeling can generate fear, and it may seem easier to stay with what is familiar than to venture into the unknown.

The extra weight also keeps us out of the game of life, providing an excuse to avoid something rather than to risk failure. With the weight, you may justify being rejected, over-looked, or disregarded as being a result of the excess weight rather than deal with the pain of not being liked, wanted, or valued.

Another reason we may keep the weight on is to generate attention, sympathy, or extra care from those around us. Instead of finding a healthier way to meet those needs, the weight provides a visible sign that we may need the help without risking rejection by asking for it. We all want to feel cared for, connected and feel a sense of belonging. The extra attention we may receive from excess weight may give others an opportunity to provide that attention while making us feel that we are being cared for.

Yet another reason why we may keep the weight on is to punish someone or to test someone's love for us. Maybe you dislike your husband's, parents, or coworkers comments, criticism, or judgment about your weight. Keeping the weight on may be your passive/aggressive way of talking back. Finally, for some of us, keeping the weight on offers a way to test our spouse's love for us, and we may feel compelled to see if the relationship can withstand the weight.

When you're overweight yet confident, loving and supportive relationships can survive almost anything. When you're negative, pessimistic, and using your weight as a testing tool, you may want to consider what the real reason is that you're putting your relationship through this test. It takes some real soul searching to look deep within and try to understand what the excess weight provides. Does it provide security, protection, an excuse to avoid a perceived failure? Whatever the reason, it's important to discover and understand why you've chosen to keep the weight on. Now try to see if you're trying to punish anyone other than yourself, if it's rational and worthy of continuing. If you discover something traumatizing or it feels too difficult for you to handle alone, get the help and support you need to get you through. You need to commit to uncovering the reason for your weight. It's the first step to doing anything to change it.

Okay. So you know you're an emotional eater, you know you're eating as a way to self-soothe and you're aware that you may have been doing this for decades. What can you do now?

You already know that staying this way is painful, uncomfortable, and discouraging, so why not change! Even if this is all you know—you've been an emotional eater for years and can't see another way to cope with unmanaged feelings—you can still change. Although I'm not suggesting it will be easy, it's absolutely possible, beneficial, and necessary for your health and well being. There are some important steps you need to take however.

The first thing you *must* do is give yourself a break. I've said this before but it's worth repeating. Food misuse is how you've trained yourself to deal with uncomfortable feelings. It's the strategy you've employed to feel safe, secure, and temporarily rid yourself of pain. Just as you'd lovingly encourage your children to find effective coping strategies, it's important to treat yourself with the same compassion.

The next thing to do is understand why you've chosen this particular behavior. What do you risk by handling emotions another way? What are you avoiding, putting off, or not handling? What are you afraid of and is it still a legitimate fear now that you're an adult? (We often hold onto childhood fears that are irrelevant to our lives today). By asking yourself these questions, you gain a greater understanding of why you do what you do, while giving yourself an opportunity to feel compassion for yourself and your attempts to feel better through emotional eating.

Next, ask yourself what it is that you really need. If you're tired, get some sleep. If you're lonely, phone a friend, or join a group. If you feel lost, get the support you need. If you're angry, clarify why and find a constructive way to solve the problem. If you're frustrated, unfulfilled, or unsatisfied, find out how you can fulfill that need. It's also helpful to ask yourself, "What does food have to do with any of these emotions?" When you can look at it objectively, you realize that food has little to do with what it is that you are truly searching for. Using food when you need a hug is like using a hammer to screw in a screw. You need to use the right tools to get the job done more efficiently and effectively in order to give yourself what you truly need.

Something else necessary is a strong conviction that this is something you can change. You will change or not based on your belief that you can. We get so used to underestimating ourselves and our abilities. But the truth is you are capable of accomplishing so much, you can change whatever it is that you don't like and you have the ability to improve your body, mind, and soul in any way you want. I always tell my kids, "Nothing really good comes easy." Anything worthwhile takes time, effort and energy. To end your struggle with emotional eating may feel like you're wresting with an alligator. While it's difficult and exhausting, the payoff is enormous. First you're showing yourself you can change in order to think, feel, and act in a way that makes you more confident and proud. Next, you're rewiring yourself to cope differently with your stress, emotions, conflict, and pain. Finally, you're showing others, your family, and yourself that you are a role model worth emulating.

WEEKLY GOAL

- If you're an emotional eater, this week's goal is for you. The first and most important step is to give yourself some nurturing compassion! Then, work on your reactions to emotional triggers. While you may be unable to control certain factors that have triggered emotional eating in the past, what you can control is your reaction. An annoying boss last week is probably still an annoying boss this week but while last week you ate to feel better, this week choose another way to deal with your frustration. This week, commit to asking yourself "what do I really want/need" when you're headed down the path of emotional eating. Know that emotional eating only feels good until the last bite, but you'll still be left with your problems along with extra weight and frustration for not finding a better way to help yourself. Commit to giving yourself what you need and be proud of your ability to change.

Chapter 15
Triggers: People, Places, Thoughts, and Feelings

Emotional eating is so complex. It is caused by many factors both in and out of our control. While we can't control others, it's important to control how we think, feel, behave, and react. When we change our reactions, we gain a greater sense of control, empowerment, and belief in ourselves. We feel better about taking our lives into our own hands and learn to nourish our body, mind, and soul in a healthier, more desirable way. A way to preplan and prevent an emotionally induced binge is to understand our triggers—the people, places, thoughts, and feelings which lead us to overeat.

Take a look at your life. There's a great chance certain people lead you to eat emotionally. The truth is, they don't force you to eat they just trigger you to overeat. Maybe it's your kids, your mother, friend, husband, coworker, or boss. The key is to identify who leads you down the emotional eating path and why. The next step is to note the places you go that may trigger a binge. Maybe passing by that bakery before running home to catch the school bus, taking the family out for pizza, or walking past the cookie aisle causes a problem for you. Finally, what thoughts and feelings trigger you to overeat? Is it when you think about your to-do list, your commitments, or your responsibilities? What about the feelings you experience such as feeling overwhelmed, afraid, discouraged, or angry? People, places, thoughts, and feelings can all serve as triggers to emotional eating. When we understand that food won't solve any of these problems, we can work towards better ways to handle our triggers.

WEEKLY GOAL

- This week, identify who or what triggers you to eat emotionally. If it's a certain person, prepare a game plan or strategy to employ when that uncomfortable feeling arises. If it's a certain place, cross the street, get out of that aisle, choose another restaurant—find any way not to be sabotaged by the trigger. If the trigger is a thought, rephrase the thought. For example: "I'll never get all of this complete" can be rephrased to "I'll do the best I can to complete what's most important." Finally, if the trigger is a feeling, know that emotionally eating will leave you with that feeling plus many more when you're finished eating. Find a way to feel better while not allowing yourself to be sabotaged by the trigger. This week, commit to identifying your triggers and stopping them from derailing you.

Chapter 16
Simple Solutions to Save Time and Pre-Plan

As we've seen so far, our relationship with food can be extremely complicated. As moms, your life is complicated enough so it's important to find ways to make your life easier. Here are some ways to make food preparation, purchasing, and pre-planning easy so you struggle with food less while allowing more time for the things you enjoy.

Studies have shown that approximately 50 percent of our food dollars are spent on restaurant eating with convenience and saving time the most popular reasons for eating outside the home. That means more eating out, take out, fast food, and dashboard dining. If we do eat at home, studies show that only 50 percent of us eat something homemade. The most popular meals eaten at home take less than a total of fifteen minutes to prepare and seven out of ten shoppers purchase prepared meals when food shopping in order to save time. We've already seen how foods can be loaded with sugar, fat, and calories when we choose to eat outside the home. Portions can be enormous and saving time is replaced with eating much more than we need. Prepared meals can also be hazardous because of the sugar, fat, preservatives, stabilizers, and fillers they may contain. In our effort to eat more healthfully while not spending our day in the kitchen, what is there to do?

One option is to make multiple portions of something, then package and freeze what you don't need for a later date. You can double a recipe for a healthy soup, low fat stew, or use an interesting grain dish. You can also use one food and prepare it in a few ways to use for other meals. For example, usually once each week I'll buy the family size portion of chicken cutlets. I'll take out a few trays and coat some cutlets with barbeque sauce, others with seasoning, and save a few to use in a stir fry. I'll prepare the chicken after I've given my kids breakfast while they're in the kitchen eating their breakfast. It provides time together where we can talk about our upcoming day while they see me using some time management skills! You can also buy precut, pre washed, and pre packaged salads and vegetables for easy use. Making a salad is easier than ever without having to cut, chop, dice, or slice.

You can also have a round table discussion of foods your family will eat (young children may not be speaking yet, but let's assume you know what they like). Find alternatives that work for all of you so that you're not making a specific meal for everyone. Many moms prepare one meal for the kids, another for their husband, and another for themselves. With many kids, we may cater to the preferences of each one giving us the job of making a multitude of meals at once! When we were kids, one meal was prepared and we found something to eat on the plate. Mom wasn't a short order cook then but has become one now. The short order cook approach makes preparing a meal exhausting and time consuming. If this is how meal preparation operates in your home, you may want to consider a more time saving (and aggravation sparing) solution.

If your budget allows, there are many other ways to save time on food shopping and preparation. Many grocery store delivery services are available today. For a fee (usually less than $10) you can do your food shopping online. Every category of food is listed and you check off the type and amount of each food that you want. Choose the delivery time and decide when it's best to receive your food. With larger families, you may find that you shop more than once or twice per week adding up to a few hours spent at the supermarket. When you add up those hours, think of what else you could be doing instead!

Another option has been popping up all over the internet. There are many services available where you list your food preferences along with how you'd like the food to be prepared (low fat, under fifteen minutes to prepare, etc.). For a fee, you receive recipes along with a pre printed shopping list allowing you to buy all of the ingredients you'll need to prepare each meal for the week or month. These services save time preparing shopping lists and looking through cookbooks or magazines for ideas while offering an interesting take on foods you already enjoy. Some interesting menus can be found at www.menuplanningcentral.com/lfi.

WEEKLY GOAL

- Do you eat out often to save time? Do you buy prepared food, takeout or fast food because it's more convenient? Are you the family's short order cook? This week, commit to trying some time saving tricks whether it's how you shop to how you prepare your foods. Think of all of the time, effort, and energy you can save in addition to all of the extra money and calories you spend while eating for convenience. The extra money you save can be spent on something fun and the calories, fat, and sugar saved can be priceless if you're struggling to get back into your pre pregnancy jeans! Commit to a time saving strategy and make it part of your healthy new way of eating.

Changing your eating habits is never an easy task. It takes leaving a comfort zone of what may provide as much comfort as those pink fuzzy slippers you've worn for years. While the slippers may feel comfortable, a great pair of heels or boots can make you feel sexier, more confident, empowered and strong. That's how taking control of your eating can make you feel. Through healthy lifestyle changes you gain a feeling of being in control by taking charge of your eating instead of letting your poor eating habits and behaviors control you. You become more aware of what triggers sabotage your best efforts and learn how to prepare for them so you stay on track. You learn that while falling off track is normal and expected, every effort needs to be made to get back on. You learn to become more mindful of your eating so every bite counts. You learn how to eat for fuel, nourishment, and enjoyment versus eating to self-soothe. You learn to make healthier choices in order to provide your body with the quality, freshness, vitamins, and minerals it deserves. You learn how to get off the detrimental diet track where all you eventually lose is your confidence, self-esteem, and belief that you can successfully lose weight. Finally, through lifestyle changes, you learn to set small, measurable goals in order to achieve long lasting results. Remember, weight loss is a journey. The more unhealthy habits you change into healthy habits, the more weight loss success you'll have. To try to lose the weight too quickly will only leave you frustrated, angry, guilty and depressed so go for progress rather than perfection. Finally, please use the special link to reach me at www.TheMojoCoach.com/contact.php because I'm eager to cheer you on when you tell me about your latest success. Hang in there. Remember, nothing really good comes easy.

Stress Control
Fitness Program

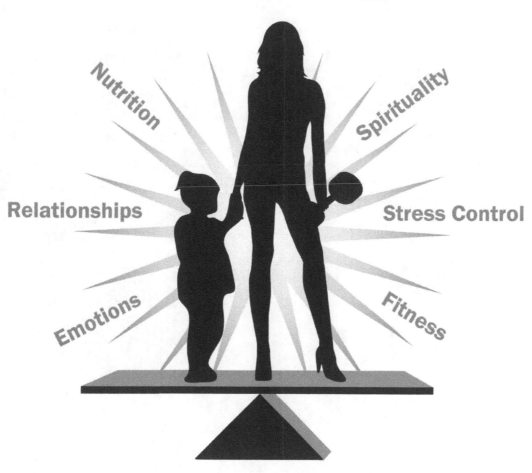

Introduction

There are two types of stress. The first type is acute stress. That's the kind where your body senses danger and adapts to the threat by making physical changes that enable you to quickly get out of harm's way. This occurs because your body secretes chemicals and stress hormones such as adrenaline and cortisol. These chemicals are secreted in response to your thoughts and cause your body to prepare for "fight or flight." For example, let's say you are crossing the street and you notice a car quickly approaching. You see the car, which causes you to feel fear and anxiety. Your body then adapts to the stress by secreting chemicals and hormones that send messages to your heart, lungs, and organs in order to prepare them to handle your crisis. Your heart rate increases, blood flow is diverted to muscles allowing for quick movement, your pupils dilate and more oxygen flows through your lungs for an extra burst of energy. These changes allow you to react quickly, enabling you to jump onto the curb to safety. Within a short period of time your body calms down and things return to normal. This protective mechanism is crucial to your safety and is designed to protect you against danger.

The other type of stress is called chronic stress. With chronic stress, chemicals and hormones that were only intended to be secreted for a short period of time are continually being released. The stress response is engaged and never turned off. Glands that secrete these chemicals don't have an opportunity to replenish or restore themselves to pre-stress levels. Your body remains in a state of hyper arousal and hormones that are meant to help and protect you are over-secreted and eventually depleted. It's like turning on the shower at full force and leaving it on. Eventually, you're going to run out of hot water.

Stress and the immune system are very closely linked. Your immune system maintains internal harmony within your body. When it is healthy and strong, it is in fighting shape to protect you against unwanted invasion. One of the biggest dangers with chronic stress is that the over-secretion of chemicals suppresses your immune system. When this occurs, your body doesn't have the ability to fight off invaders as effectively, so you have less protection against illness, stress related conditions, and disease. The immune system is directly affected by the way we handle stress. If it's strong, it offers us protection, if it is weak, it is unable to fight for us:(Have you ever noticed how you may get a respiratory infection when you're under a lot of stress? The stress you were under caused a release of hormones, which weakened your immune system and couldn't protect you against the invader).

Stress hormones and chemicals are released according to the way we think, feel and act. The way we think, feel and act is based on our ideas, beliefs, value system, religious upbringing, personality, culture, and past conditioning. All of these variables determine how we are affected by stress because they create how we view the world around us. One event can be viewed so differently by two people depending on their perspective. For example, have you ever noticed how two people can view traffic? One person can be seen banging their steering wheel, cursing, and drowning in a sea of stress induced hormones. The other person can be seen catching up on phone calls, listening to music, and enjoying a quiet moment for themselves. It's the same event for both, but how the event is regarded is completely different and is based on the way each one interprets the event. While we are all affected by stress differently, people who are better equipped to handle the stressors in their lives are the ones who enjoy the greatest health and wellness benefits. Their bodies aren't continually releasing stress hormones that cause immune system damage along with other bodily wear and tear.

When these chemicals are being constantly secreted, over time they can also cause stress induced conditions, illness, and disease because they alter the chemistry of your cells while weakening your immune system. When hormones such as cortisol are depleted, autoimmune diseases can occur and conditions like arthritis are common. When levels are abnormal, other problems arise. Sleep quality, skin disorders, infertility, anxiety, and delayed healing are all common when stress hormones are out of balance.

Stress also affects the nervous system which is directly tied to the digestive system. Ever notice how you many feel gassy, bloated or like you haven't fully digested when you scarf down lunch? Your body interpreted the stress you were feeling and decided that it was more important to prepare you for the perceived battle than to effectively digest your meal. Digestive disturbances are so widespread that they are now the largest emergency room complaint. Conditions like reflux, Chrohn's disease, irritable bowel syndrome, and ulcers are all so common and can all be tied to stress.

If things weren't bad enough, stress also causes us to age more quickly. This happens when cortisol is over secreted. There isn't enough and more needs to be produced. Levels are regained by borrowing chemicals from your estrogen stores, but those are needed to help retain youth and vitality. Have you even noticed someone and thought "Wow, that person looks like they've had a hard life." The way they've handled their stress is written all over them.

When you thought things couldn't get worse, stress can also make you overweight! Here's what happens. When you're stressed, the stress hormones are released and increase your appetite for high fat, high calorie foods. You then eat those foods, and those are the foods that encourage the release of stress hormones!

It's an endless cycle leading to the over-secretion of stress hormones, weight gain, and frustration. These hormones also encourage fat to be stored in your abdominal region, increase the amount of glucose floating around in your blood, and lay the groundwork for insulin resistance, diabetes, high cholesterol, and hypertension. So, the stress you interpret encourages you to eat foods that make you heavier which then causes the release of more chemicals. If you're an emotional eater, you're in even bigger trouble.

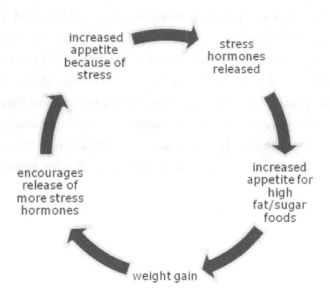

Now you've added extra eating as way to self-medicate to feel better from your stress. You may choose foods high in fat and sugar that gives you a boost of the feel good chemical serotonin. This lifts you up but then drops you hard and you are left with less energy than before.

At this point, you're left with your original stress, the feelings regarding your eating habits, the excess weight—a starting point for illness or disease—and stress hormones on a rampage.

It's important to realize that the stress response was designed to be effective when used for short term safety. Unfortunately, those same chemicals that protect you from immediate danger hurt you when they continue to be released. To make matters worse, the body doesn't know if the stress is real or merely imagined. It will secrete stress hormones whether you're grieving over the death of a loved one, reacting to your kids making you crazy, or replaying the pain, hurt, or argument you had with your mother ten years ago.

We often don't realize how the stress we feel can lead to a physical response. It may be easier to accept that a physical response is due to a physical cause. For example, you stub your toe, you scream out in pain. But think of this. You hear something embarrassing or something that makes you angry. The message is heard and interpreted by you according to the way you've learned to think, feel, and act. As a result, you blush or even turn beet red! If you're nervous about something, you may feel "butterflies" or your hands may get clammy. If you're angry you may feel "your blood boil," you may have a "sour stomach," or you may feel heat coming off of you. All of these examples are physical reactions to emotions. The message was heard, interpreted, chemicals were secreted and you had a physical reaction to the message. That's just one incidence! Now imagine the stress of motherhood, trying to be a good wife, coworker, daughter, sister, friend, or neighbor. Add the need to be perfect, liked, approved, admired, and respected. Mix it with the stress, strain, and anxiety of past hurts, grievances, and negative feelings stemming from a perspective that doesn't serve you well. What have you got? A recipe for stress related conditions, illness, and disease. While this may seem frightening, the beauty is you are in a wonderful position to stop the stress response. Remember, your stress may not change. What can change, however, is the way you choose to react to it.

Chapter 1
Identifying Your Stress

N ow that I've made you significantly more stressed than you already were, I'll give you some helpful tips on how to reduce your stress level so you are in a better position to minimize stress related conditions. The more information you have, the more you can understand yourself and see why you think, feel, and act the way you do. When you understand yourself better, you can shape, sculpt, and redirect your thinking so you can become more "stress hardy" (a term coined by researcher Dr. Suzanne Kobassa).

Someone who is "stress hardy" doesn't experience any less stress than you do. They may not have easier, saner, or more comfortable lives than you. What they do have however is a higher threshold for stress. With a higher threshold for stress, they have a higher tolerance and can cope with stress more effectively without releasing a cascade of stress hormones. A person with a high tolerance for stress is committed to themselves, their health, happiness, and their well being. They know they need to show themselves some self-care in order to be ready, willing, and able to deal with stress within their lives. They feel a sense of control over their lives as well. They control their lives rather than allowing life to control them. They realize that their thoughts, beliefs, and actions put them in the position they're in and they are directly controlling where they are, what they think, and where they're going. A person with a high stress tolerance is also able to embrace challenges that come their way. For these people, change is seen as a challenge to embrace rather than something to run from.

A recent study by the American Psychological Association found that women were more affected by stress than men and report engaging in behaviors such as emotional eating, poor diet choices, smoking, and inactivity in an effort to deal with their stress. Unmanaged stress is so detrimental to your health that it can contribute to the onset of disease, worsen symptoms of an existing disease or cause a relapse of a previous illness or condition. A large portion of this stress occurs when we juggle too many things, take too much on, over promise, over commit, and over extend ourselves. What's going on here?

A recent study also found that there is a common theme found in people who suffer the most from the affects of chronic stress. These people live a lifestyle where their work and finances are always a major concern. They don't get adequate amounts of sleep, which is necessary to renew and replenish the body. Their diets are of poor quality. They are eating high sugar, high fat, nutrient-void, calorie-dense "sub foods." They don't have adequate stress control outlets in the form of exercise, meditation, yoga, visualization, gardening, etc. Finally, they view their lives from a victim perspective. They don't feel they have any control over the lives they live or the cards they've been dealt and see no way things could change for the better. Many of these characteristics can be applied to many moms today. Juggling responsibilities, commitments, and the schedules of everyone in her care leaves no time, energy, or motivation to add something else to juggle—the need for self-care.

If this sounds like you or if you see any similar characteristics to your own it's time to get your stress under control. Before you can implement a game plan to reduce your stress level, you need to identify the *who, what, when, where, how,* and *why* of stress.

This means, you first need to understand *who* brings on your stress. Is it your children, your husband, your parents, siblings, or coworkers? Why do you feel more stressed because of them and what are they doing or saying that makes you feel the way you do? Next you need to determine under *what* circumstances do you feel stressed. Is it when you're rushed, pressured with a deadline, at a specific time in your day? Are you leaving yourself enough time to handle a specific task or would factoring in an extra fifteen or twenty minutes help you to prepare yourself? After that, discover *when* it is that you are most likely to experience feelings of stress. Is it when you compare yourself to other moms, before a particular type of social event, when going about your daily responsibilities or commitments? Do you feel that the stress you're feeling by the person, place, or event is justified?

Next note *how* your body reacts to the stress. Do you feel your heart racing, body getting warmer, breathing becoming quick and shallow? Does it feel physically uncomfortable to you and do you notice the difference in how you feel when you're relaxed, calm and breathing deeply and slowly? Finally, determine *why* you are reacting to stress the way you do. Did you take on too much or over commit? Do you feel others will be disappointed if you are unable to accomplish it all? If you choose to do less in order to feel less stressed do you feel inadequate, insecure or incapable? If so, where did these feelings originate and do they make sense today?

I asked you a lot of questions because the more you know about yourself, the better you can design an effective plan to manage your stress. The better armed you are with knowledge, the better armed you'll be to effectively curtail your stress before incurring too much damage. Now that you've asked yourself all of these questions, this goal's for you.

WEEKLY GOAL

- Take the time to find the answers to the questions above. Identify each of these factors to understand your personal response and reactions to the stressors within your life. Find out the types of situations that most greatly affect you and learn how your body specifically interprets the stress you feel. Most importantly, please understand that you don't have to respond the way you do even though that's what you've always been doing. If it doesn't work, that's exactly why it needs to be changed! You're an adult now. The way you handle, control and manage your stress needs to be specifically designed by you and for you. If the path you've taken with regards to stress is causing you to feel frazzled, out of control and unhappy, it's not the best plan for you and make gradual changes in order to make it better. Once you understand how *you* operate, you are in a better place to change your view. This week, commit to finding out your personal who, what, when, where, how, and why regarding stress. You'll need a total of six answers, one each for who, what, when, where, how, and why. Write each answer down if it helps you to visually see your stress triggers. The better you understand your triggers, the better you can handle, manage, or avoid them.

Chapter 2
Stress and Sleep

Studies have found that 75–90 percent of all doctor visits are related to stress. Stress can show itself in many ways, from anxiety, irritability, intolerance, and frustration to difficulty focusing, extreme fatigue, and insomnia. It's a Catch-22 when it comes to stress and sleep. The body requires sleep to more effectively deal with the affects of stress but the stress you feel reduces the ability to get enough sleep.

In order to function adequately, your body requires seven to eight hours of sleep per night. Without adequate sleep, we're left feeling irritable, cranky, short fused, emotionally unstable, mentally cloudy, groggy, fatigued—and overweight. This happens because when we're sleep deprived, stress hormones are released, which disrupt the normal rhythm of our sleep cycle. Instead of waking feeling refreshed, high cortisol levels leave you feeling groggy and fatigued. If that weren't bad enough, this high cortisol level that is released during times of little sleep also increases our appetite for high fat, high sugar foods. In addition, when we're tired, we look for ways to increase our energy. One way is by taking in simple carbohydrates and the other is by taking in caffeine.

Taking in simple carbohydrates (sugar) for your energy boost is one of the easiest ways to gain weight. The calories add up quickly, you're never full or satisfied, and the sugar you're taking in simply encourages the intake of more refined sugar. (Other problems associated with a high sugar intake can be found in the Nutritional Fitness Program Section).

While many of us use sugar as a quick energy boost, many of us use caffeine in an effort to wake up. Here's what happens when you're looking for energy through caffeine. For some, you may feel nervous, anxious and shaky. Also, while you may have an additional energy boost from the caffeine, if the body needs rest and has caffeine instead, you'll have that feeling of being "tired and wired." You may be able to get through your day, but this artificial energy takes you further away from readjusting to a healthy, balanced sleep cycle. The stress hormones have no opportunity to replenish and the body experiences immune system damage along with physical, mental, and emotional wear and tear.

Now I could tell you to make sure you get those hours in and settle for nothing less, but those of you with young children may not have this luxury just yet. If you are doing late night feedings, your child is having nightmares, night terrors, or he or she is having difficulty staying asleep, the idea of a full night's sleep may seem priceless but not possible at this time. For you, the best option may be to nap when and if you can. Catching even fifteen or twenty minutes somewhere in your day can do wonders to refuel and recharge your body.

Although seven to eight hours of sleep is preferred, there are a few strategies you can try to make whatever sleep you can get more effective. First, limit your caffeine and try not to have anything caffeinated in the afternoon. The caffeine that may help get you through your afternoon will discourage restful sleep later on. Coffee, tea, soda, and chocolate all contain caffeine so use with discretion.

This next strategy has to do with putting yourself in the best mental position for sleep. Many of my clients have found it extremely helpful to write things down or talk things out before going to sleep. Once your thoughts, ideas, and concerns are "on the table" you may be better able to relax. You may feel you don't have to think about them anymore because they've been somewhat dealt with.

Sleep experts have also found that a sleep routine is helpful. That means trying to go to sleep at the same time, making the room dark and cool, playing soft music or "white noise," maybe taking a warm bath and making your bedroom clean, serene, and comfortable. A messy room or leaving paperwork sitting around may remind you of all you need to do and may cause you to feel stress. Having your bedroom "sleep ready" can give you a better chance to get some quality sleep. Are you doing all you can to prepare yourself for a good night's sleep? If not, here's this week's goal.

WEEKLY GOAL

- We have two goals here. One is about getting your body ready for sleep and the other is for getting the room ready for quality sleep. Let's start with you. This week, commit to no caffeine after 1:00 p.m. or 2:00 p.m., write things down, talk them through, and do whatever you can to lay down with a clear head. Tell yourself you're "clocking out" and can think of everything you have to do once you wake up. Give yourself the best opportunity possible for quality sleep by preparing your body and your mind. The second goal is preparing your room so it's a place of serenity and calm. How are the colors? Are they vibrant and stimulating? Maybe consider some calming colors that soothe you. There are so many aromatherapy candles, oils, etc. with calming scents like lavender to calm your senses as well. Music, white noise, reading before bed may also be some ideas to try. Experiment in order to design an atmosphere that encourages you to feel calm and relaxed. This week it's all about preparing your room and yourself for quality sleep.

Chapter 3
Super Mom

There are a few battles constantly waging war within most moms. The battles are due to self-imposed, unrealistic standards we've designed for ourselves. While we may feel good when we meet these high standards, they cause enormous amounts of stress and falling short leaves us with filled with blame, doubt and insecurity. Here are a few examples.

What is your idea of a good mom? Is it a woman who always looks great, never loses her cool, and manages her home, business, family, and self with ease and perfection? Are her kids always neat, bright, and well behaved, her house always spotless, her style always cutting edge? Is she always made up, with perfect hair, nails, and toes? How about her husband, is he charming, involved, and successful? Who came up with all this and what benefit could it possibly give us by finding fault with ourselves if we have anything less? It's great to set high standards for yourself and your family and of course you want the best of everything. That being said, although it's possible to have it all, sometimes it's just not possible to have it all *at the same time*.

With young, messy kids running through your house, it may not be the best time to expect your home to look like a museum. When you haven't slept in days, you may not feel like spending the extra energy to prepare a five course meal and maybe something simpler will do.

When you just delivered your baby, it may not be the best time to berate yourself for not being able to button the pre-pregnancy jeans. I'm not saying these things can't and won't happen they may just not happen the minute you want them to and that's okay. What can you do?

The first and most important thing to do is take some pressure off yourself. Realize these expectations and standards are self-imposed and causing you mental, physical, and emotional stress (and you know what *that* stress can do). You decided these standards were important so you're the one who needs to decide they don't work for you anymore. By relaxing unrealistic expectations you'll take some of the pressure off that's been a great source of stress. Come to grips with the idea that with a plan, you'll get to it all in time.

The next thing to do is prioritize what is important to you. For example, let's say healthy eating and exercising are your most immediate concerns. If that's something you feel needs your attention, make the decision to spend the time planning your meals, cooking more healthfully, and exercising while loosening up your standards about having a spotless house and go for neat instead. Lose the guilt and let it go! If your children need extra attention in order to behave in a more socially acceptable way, spend the time on them and cut back somewhere else like surfing the net or watching TV. If you've been neglecting your relationships, cut back somewhere else and find the time to connect. Without a plan, it's easy to allow stress to paralyze and consume you. This leaves us feeling powerless and without hope. There are only so many hours in a day so it's important to schedule your day with your priorities in mind. Schedule them into your calendar or date book like an appointment. Make no excuses, feel good about your decision and honor your schedule the best way you can. It's time for a goal.

WEEKLY GOAL

- Look at your schedule. Decide what needs to change, where you can relax your standards and where you can incorporate something beneficial. Changing everything at once causes you to feel stressed so choose one area where you'll loosen up in order to find the time for something more important to you at this time. Make your decision and be confident about it whether it involves your own self-care, your family, your relationships, your home, work, whatever. Commit to incorporating what's important while eliminating the stress, anguish, and frustration you may feel by not having everything "perfect." Remember, you can be great at everything, just not all at the same time.

I'll give you an example. I have a husband, four children, four dogs, a home, and a business. While many things are important to me, it's just not realistic or feasible to expect things to be perfect all the time or expect that I'll be the one able to do it all. To preserve my sanity and well being, certain things needed to go. I enlisted the support of some very good friends to help keep me on track with things that weren't an immediate priority to me.

For example, I have one friend who loves to shop. I hate to shop and would rather do almost anything else, so she provides me with a crucial service. She tells me exactly when I need to go to the stores and buy the end of the season clothes at half price in order to have my kids ready for the following season without spending a ton of money. When I get the call, no thinking is required. I simply respond like a robot and purchase everything necessary in the next size up.

Another friend is a master organizer. When we celebrate anyone's birthday, she figures out everyone's schedules in order to make a reservation at a restaurant, handles the purchase of the card and gift and even coordinates a carpool so we can all ride together. I simply ask "what time do I need to be ready" and "how much do I owe."

Find out where you could use some help and simply…ASK for it. While it may be difficult at first, you'll quickly realize how powerful and how useful this simple tip can be.

Chapter 4
Micromanaging and Delegating

Feeling a sense of control is important to your health, self-esteem and well being. It helps us feel strong, empowered and in charge of our lives and the way it's unfolding. While a sense of control is beneficial, too much control often leaves us micromanaging everything and everyone in our path. Are you micromanaging? Do you need to oversee everything and make sure it's all done your way? Is it unsettling for you when things aren't done to your exact specifications? Besides taking on an enormous amount of extra stress, you're probably annoying everyone in your path. If this sounds like you, it's time to stop micromanaging, delegate, and let go. First of all, consider it from your children's perspective.

Let's say you ask them to make their bed. The cover may be pulled up but it's not tucked in with military precision by any means. You've asked them to handle the bed making task, it doesn't meet your approval so you decide to remake their bed. What message are your children receiving while you're satisfying your need for a perfect house? They're probably feeling like their efforts aren't good enough, which discourages them from trying harder while diminishing their self-esteem. Here's another example.

You've asked your husband to go food shopping in an effort to share the workload—so far, so good. He comes home with every concoction of sugary, fatty junk food that can be found on the supermarket shelves. What do you do? Maybe you play martyr and decide that he can't get it right so it's just another job you'll have to do. You pout and storm away. Who are you punishing here? Yes you'll bring home some healthier options, but how about providing him with a specific list and hoping for the best? Your first option only leaves you with more work, frustration, and unhappiness while he's off the hook and wishing you could simply ask for what you want.

The trick with ending micromanaging is to delegate the task and then let it go! Sure it may not be perfect or exactly the way you want it. But I'm going to ask you a very deep, spiritual, and philosophical question that can only be answered after careful though and consideration. Ready, the question is—who cares? Chances are no one cares but you. Delegating a task frees you up for something better and usually more rewarding. Unfortunately, however, many of us are afraid to let go for a few reasons.

Some of us are afraid to give up control by leaving tasks to others and the only way to reduce the fear is by retaining control. We may hesitate to let go because we're insecure about the outcome without our interference or may only feel comfortable if things are done our way and on our terms.

Some of us may not want to spend the money on delegating certain responsibilities and feel that the money saved justifies the extra work. For example, maybe you can easily afford to hire a babysitter once a week in order to go out with your husband at night or take care of some errands more quickly during the day. You determine how much you'd need to spend on the babysitter and determine it's not worth the price. "I'll just go out with my husband another time or drag the kids along on my errands." The money you save by not hiring the babysitter may not cost nearly as much as the price you pay by neglecting your relationships and dragging your kids away from happily playing at home.

Still some of us fear the judgment they'll receive if they delegate certain responsibilities to someone else. Here's the "super mom" syndrome again. Maybe you fear people will talk if you get help cleaning the house, hiring a babysitter, or having someone help you with a task you'd rather not do. By delegating, you're freeing yourself up to do something you find more valuable, fulfilling, and necessary. By doing the task because you fear judgment you are wasting valuable time that could be spent on something you'd enjoy much more. I'll give you a personal example.

When my youngest son was in his last year of preschool, I was scheduling work appointments around his schedule in order for me to be able to drive him to and from his school that was less than two miles away. I purposely worked from home so I could work around my children's schedules, but his preschool hours required that I not schedule two appointments each day just so I could take him to and from school. We spent time in the morning before school (his day started after my three other children's day so we had time alone together) and I was completely available to him once his school day was over. I felt satisfied with the amount and quality of time we spent.

I was told of this great new service that provided transportation to school and was specifically designed for children. Children's music filled the car, toys were in baskets in the van and it was a great way for the children to leave their homes and feel like big kids on their own "special bus" before getting on a bus for Kindergarten.

How would it look if my son went to school in this decorated minivan just so I could work? What would the other moms think if my son didn't have me to hold his hand before he walked into his class? Was I a bad mom and was I choosing work over my child? After torturing myself adequately, I decided that the best way to determine what was best for me was by having a "meeting" with my son. Here's how it went: "Cole, you know that minivan you see at school with all the writing on the outside? That minivan can take you to and from school, but if they do, mommy won't be driving you. What I will do is put you on the bus in the morning and be waiting to take you off the bus when you come home. What do you think?"

"Yeah!" he says. "Our car just has yucky stuff in it. The van has the best toys, my friends all told me!" The decision was made and everyone was happy. As far as being judged by the other moms, here's what I figured. They'll probably judge me no matter what I do, so I might as well do what's best for me and my family. Besides, if they're judging me, do I really want to be friends with them anyway? I then asked myself my deep, spiritual question…who cares?! So for your health, well being, and sanity, it's time for a goal.

WEEKLY GOAL

- Are you micromanaging? Do you always have to have control and feel only your way is best? If so, commit to one area where you can delegate and let go. If it's having the kids clean their rooms, delegate the job, close the door and let it go! If your husband has yet to perfect the art of changing a diaper, wish him luck and let it go! If your child thinks his school project is perfect, bite your tongue, put your hands in your pockets so you can't fix it and let it go! Commit to one area to delegate and let go. You'll be amazed at how easy it becomes once you get the hang of it and how much free time and mental space you have as a result.

Chapter 5
Organizing: De-Cluttering Your Space to De-Clutter Your Mind

L ook around you. Don't just glance, take a good look around. What do you see? Your surroundings reflect how you feel and you can learn a lot about your internal environment by looking at your external environment. For example, do you work or live in a space that's messy and uncared for? If so there's a good chance that you feel messy and uncared for yourself. Is your environment disorganized, cluttered, and confusing? You may be feeling that same way yourself. Your surroundings are either supportive or destructive to your well being. They can either enhance and soothe or unnerve and distress you. If they don't work for you, it's time to organize your space, which will help organize your life. It's time to de-clutter your space in order to de-clutter your mind, which will lead to greater focus and clarity. It's time to get your living and working space organized, clutter free, and calm. You can also get additional help from organizations and websites designed to help you become clutter free.

Organizing your space is a proactive way to support a healthy lifestyle. It brings about a sense of serenity that simply feels good. It makes life less distracting because it eliminates the constant reminder and mental burden that comes with staring at an unfinished task. It frees up space and time to pursue something enriching, satisfying and fulfilling. It gives you a greater sense of control, accomplishment, and confidence in a goal set and achieved. Finally, it helps you find things more easily!

Let's start with de-cluttering your space. It's important to de-clutter first so you don't organize things you don't intend to keep. Go into your closet. Do you still have clothes from the 1980's? Are you still hanging onto your shoulder-padded blazers and snake-skin mini skirt? The basic rule here is "when in doubt, throw it out." Never ride a fashion trend twice and strive to look the best you can—for your age. Pack the stuff in bags, donate the clothes to charity or host a "clothes swapping party" where friends bring their bags of clothes and you can trade if you find something interesting. You'll feel so much better with the free space; you'll see what you have and be in a better position to determine what items you need. Besides doing a service for yourself, you're helping others in need, which is a win-win.

The next places to tackle are your drawers, counters, and desk tops. Everything needs to have a place. Store things in specific places, label boxes with similar items, put things away, not down. Start by sorting items into piles to file, store, keep, or toss. Then keep what's important, discard what's not, store and file the rest away. Ask yourself "do I really need this and will I notice or mind if it's gone?" If the answer is no, throw it out. Also, tie up some loose ends by determining if something broken is worth fixing such as electronic equipment in need of repair and clothing that needs to be altered or fixed. These unfinished tasks are vying for your attention and are causing mental distraction. So if it's worth it, fix it immediately. If it's not, toss it out.

It's also important to realize that small steps add up and you need not overhaul everything all at once. To make a dent in your de-clutter plan, one option is to set a timer for ten or fifteen minutes each time you de-clutter. Just by devoting a small amount of time each day can make a difference over the course of a few weeks. Whatever the task you're focusing on for the day, set the timer and go! Don't forget to celebrate your efforts because whatever you got to during that time is more than you would have gotten to without trying at all.

You can focus on organizing your garage, pantry, or car as well. Put up hooks to utilize wall space, use clear plastic bins to see and store items easily, and use hanging clear shoe bags placed on the back of a door to organize supplies that would get lost in a drawer. Discard your junk mail, old medicine, makeup, and unidentifiable objects sitting in the back of your refrigerator. Respond to those overdue calls or emails, and put your bills, receipts and important papers in order. Any area where you de-clutter and organize will bring you a sense of completion, pride, and calm.

This next tip is for when you have a "pack rat" in the family. I often hold a "thumb up, thumb down party" with my kids. They sit on their beds and with a big garbage bag in hand, I go through their drawers and look for a thumbs-up or thumbs-down. Thumbs-up means they want to keep the item; thumbs-down means they don't care if I throw it away. It's a task that enables us to spend time and have fun. I get to de-clutter, and they can't complain that they're working so hard. The other trick when you have a pack rat is to store things away when your pack rat isn't looking. After a few months without them even realizing the item was missing, casually mention that you put it away. Nine times out of ten they realize they don't need it anymore, never missed it, and don't care what you do with it.

Once there is a greater sense of order, it's helpful to organize the rest of your surroundings to give yourself a sense of structure and control. Many of my clients have found it beneficial to write lists or write down important thoughts as a way to stay more organized. Studies have found that thoughts can be lost from your memory in a matter of seconds if they're not written down, so keeping a list is a great way to stay on top of things. One tip that's always worked for me is posting my children's schedules on the inside of their closed door. They can check the day (with your help if they can't read) and see how they need to dress or what they need to bring depending on their individual schedule.

If it helps reduce your stress, prepare for a busy day the night before, organize important paperwork, pick out clothes, prepare lunches and snacks for your kids before leaving the kitchen at night, or leave things by the front door so you make sure to take them with you. By becoming more organized, you become less stressed because you've freed up mental space and energy to pursue what you enjoy. You spend less time searching for lost items, feeling rushed, anxious, and harried because there is a place for everything and everything is in its place. De-cluttering and organizing can also be helpful tools if timeliness or procrastination is an issue for you.

Are you always running late, frantically trying to get somewhere on time, or constantly apologizing because you just couldn't get to where you needed to be when you needed to be there? Getting your space in order is a great way to help better manage your time for many reasons. When you're more organized, you know where you can find what you need. In a de-cluttered space you have less mental distractions and you're better able to focus on the task at hand. Finally, the sense of accomplishment you feel from organizing your space gives you a sense of appreciation for yourself and overflows to those around you. As you begin to appreciate yourself and your surroundings it's natural to want to show others this same appreciation and respect. Timeliness is a way to show your respect for someone else's time. It shows that you value them, their schedule and their commitments as you value and respect your own.

When you organize and de-clutter, you are helping to end your battle with procrastination. We procrastinate when we don't want to do something, fear we won't do it well, or risk failure at a job poorly done. Once your space is uncluttered and your life more organized as a result, certain tasks don't need to be put off because they aren't as insurmountable. If I asked you to walk from New York to California, you'd call me crazy and say it can't be done because you consider it an insurmountable task. If I simply told you to put one foot in front of the other, day after day, and carefully kept you on the correct path, eventually, although you'd be very tired, you'd get there. The point is we can do anything when it's broken down into bite sized chunks and it's a formula that can keep the desire to procrastinate at bay.

When you de-clutter your space, you bring about a sense of calm, serenity, and pride. This reduces your stress, enhances your confidence, and gives you an opportunity to be more peaceful and relaxed. If you're feeling cluttered, unorganized, or you're constantly running late, this goal's for you.

WEEKLY GOAL

■ It's important to take it slowly here. Depending on your surroundings, de-cluttering may seem like an overwhelming task so it's best to start small. Start with one drawer, one area or one room at a time. Celebrate your new found space and feel the sense of accomplishment at a job well done. Enjoy the greater sense of peace you feel with your new space. This week, commit to de-clutter. Start with organizing your pictures into a photo album, a desk drawer, junk drawer, or whatever can use your immediate attention first.

Chapter 6
No, Yes, and Should

No, yes, and should are probably three of the most stressful and misused words that we use today. They create an enormous amount of stress, anxiety, and pressure when used inappropriately. Let's start with the word yes. So often we say yes to something when our body, heart, and soul are screaming *no!!!* Have you ever been asked to do something that you knew would be a huge undertaking, zap you of all of your energy, freedom, and time? Every ounce of you wanted to decline the offer in order to preserve your best interests. You may have hesitated, wavered, hemmed and hawed, but within a short period of time you said yes. Maybe you felt it was the only option you had in order to be accepted, be viewed as a "good mom," prove you were a team player, or show your value to the person or group. Once you said "yes," however, you felt overburdened, taken advantage of, and wished you had listened to that inner voice of reason that was gently prodding you to say no. Why is it so hard to say no?

Many of us find saying no extremely painful and difficult. Fear, doubt, and their cousin, insecurity, are often the powerful forces that render us incapable of saying no. But look at it this way. As difficult as it may be for you to say no, the downside is much worse. The few minutes of discomfort when that person expects you to say yes and you decline can be excruciating. But that exchange only lasts a few minutes and the freedom you've secured lasts much longer. By saying no you've also stayed true to yourself and your values. Let's say you feel you've been shortchanging your husband, children, or friends by not having any free time for them. Saying no to another commitment frees you up to give them your quality time. You're preserving what's important to you and reminding yourself of that can give you the strength to just say no.

So often we are afraid of rejecting or offending someone and neglect to say no in order to spare the other person from these feelings. But saying no doesn't mean you are saying no to the person, you are simply saying no to the request. For us to assume the person has personalized and internalized the request is something we've decided for ourselves and it very often is not the case. We also associate the word yes with being nice. To overburden, overtax, and over commit yourself is not a way of showing how nice you are at all and it is worth changing this mindset. The message it does relay to those around you and yourself is how unimportant you view your own priorities, self preservation, and self care.

Now, if you realize you need to put your foot down somewhere but don't know how to start, there are gentle ways to get your message across. You may feel more comfortable buying time in order to think it through. For you, maybe "I'll have to think about it and get back to you" is the way to go. If no time is needed to think about it, you want to ensure the person knows for certain the answer is a no and you want to stop being the usual "go to" person, you may want to consider another option. How about "thanks for the offer but I don't want to over-commit," "I'd love to but there's too much on my plate right now" or "now's not a good time for me. I'll let you know when I can help." Saying no doesn't make you selfish, mean, or unhelpful. It enables you to give yourself and others what is truly needed at the time.

Now let's talk about saying yes. Here's where you want to do, try, or have something. You crave it, know it will make you happy and want to include it in your life. Maybe it's buying something whimsical, pursuing a more fulfilling career, thinking "outside the box," or just doing something silly. There's that inner voice again giving you all the signs to say yes but what do you do? You say no! You think you're too old, too heavy, and not ready physically, mentally or emotionally. You believe you may not be talented, capable, or committed enough to see things through. So you turn down the offer, idea, or dream and sit with your wishes unmet and dream unfulfilled. Taking the leap is fearful, maybe terrifying and it stops you cold. This is definitely a case of yes and no confusion.

I want you to ask yourself something. Ask yourself, "What is the worst thing that can happen?" Will saying yes cause you grave illness or disease? Probably not but turning down an incredible opportunity, a chance at gratification, fulfillment, or satisfaction will leave you feeling resentful, discouraged, and unhappy. Those feelings are strong negative emotions and that's what triggers the chronic stress response.

Now think about your kids and a challenge they may face. What would you tell them? What if your son wanted to try out for a team but he may not make it. Would you tell him not to bother? What if your daughter wanted to make a new friend at preschool but she may be rejected. Would you discourage her from trying? I bet you'd tell your kids to go for it. You may even ask them "what's the worst thing that could happen?" Sure, things might not go as planned. Your son may not make the team and your daughter may need to find another friend. But by taking the chance, making the leap and giving yourself an opportunity to say yes, the results can be both rewarding and priceless.

Now let's talk about should. Should is a word filled with judgment. How does anyone know what you should do? You are the only one who knows what you should do. People offer their judgment based on their beliefs, experiences, expectations, and prior conditioning. Their thoughts are based on their perceptions which are based on how they view life and the world around them. It is within that context that they are offering you a "should." Most often it is well intentioned but very often, it causes stress and anxiety if it isn't in line with your idea at the time. What do you do with a "should" type person?

Many of us take a "should" as if it were a law. We have little faith in our own knowledge or ability and assume anyone knows better than we do. If this is how you feel, determine why you have such little faith in yourself. Are previously conditioned beliefs keeping you trapped into thinking you can't possibly know better? Are you so used to doubting yourself that you refuse to trust in your abilities? Are you so used to underestimating your talents and overestimating your faults? Chances are it's a big fat yes. For some reason, we disregard the positives and focus on the negatives. Ten positive statements about you can be negated with one negative and we don't help ourselves either. We buy into the negative like it's the truth even though it undermines our self-esteem and confidence. When this happens, someone else telling us we "should" do something seems like the only way to go. It's easier to trust them because we have lost the ability to trust ourselves. What can we do?

How about a little belief in yourself and your abilities? You have everything you need within you but as long as you doubt yourself, your talents and abilities will stay securely hidden. As long as that happens, you'll be following everyone else's "shoulds" but your own. Please understand, many people have great advice, and if it works for you by all means find a way to work it in. That's learning, growing, and evolving. But when you follow the direction of someone else because of your own self-doubt or lack of confidence you're reinforcing that doubt. Imagine a muscle. It gets stronger with use and slackens with a lack of use. Your confidence is like a muscle. When you trust yourself, you build your confidence like you're building a muscle. It strengthens each time you use it. When you don't trust yourself, you aren't strengthening the confidence muscle and it becomes weak. *Should* we have a goal? I believe so.

WEEKLY GOAL

- Think about when you say yes, no, or should. Are you saying yes when your body, heart, and soul wants to say no? Are you saying no when saying yes could bring you joy and fulfillment? Are you giving in to the judgment or demands of someone else's "should?" If so, it's time to get the right words out at the right time. This week, listen to your inner voice. If you have a feeling you'd be better off saying no, trust yourself, find a phrase that works for you, and just say no. If you've been questioning something and a lack of confidence, self-esteem, motivation, or belief in yourself has held you back, once again listen to that inner voice. It's telling you to say yes in the only way it can. By the way, that little inner voice is the only "should" you ever really need to listen to.

Chapter 7
Balance, Balance, Balance

Have you ever seen two children riding on a see-saw? It can be very interesting to watch depending on who is on either side. For example, if there is a large ten year old on one side of the see-saw and a small five year old on the other, the ten year old will be sitting on the ground, grumbling and saying how bored he is because the see-saw will not lift up. The five year old will probably be either panicking from the extreme lift off or wondering when and how she will ever get back down again. Now, imagine two average sized seven year olds. They can be seen happily giggling, enjoying the ride and the experience. They are doing what's appropriate for them, they are able to balance the see-saw because their weight is evenly distributed and they are finding joy in their experience. The point is, when the see-saw is out of balance it will not work properly and if it doesn't work it's just not fun.

Look at your life the same way using the same see-saw example. On one side, place your work, your responsibilities, your commitments, projects, tasks, your obligations, and the stress you feel from it all on one side of the see-saw. At this point you'll see that the see-saw is extremely heavy on one side and is far from balanced.

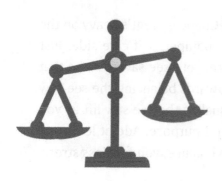

What's interesting though is that this is how many moms live their lives. The weight of one side of the see-saw is completely out of proportion with the weight on the other side. Just as the unevenly matched children were unhappy with this lack of balance, so are most moms. But while the mismatched children will quickly find a solution to make the see-saw more fun, most moms act as if there is no other alternative and keep their see-saws exactly as is. This approach leaves things terribly out of balance and simply not working.

Now go back to your see-saw and imagine what it would take to bring it into balance. First you can add some down time and enjoy it with music, taking a bath, reading a book, writing in a journal, meditating, visualizing or trying some deep breathing exercises. Maybe the see-saw budged a little bit. Now add a little bit of self care by finding time for exercise, eating well, getting more sleep, enjoying time with your family or pets, pursuing an interest and having a good laugh with your friends. See the see-saw start to lift? Continue to add a little pampering by finding time for a manicure, getting an overdue haircut, buying a new outfit or a great pair of shoes. The see-saw is lifting off and is much better balanced than before.

Each time you implement something pleasurable onto your see-saw it helps bring your life into balance. Joyful activities enable the see-saw to take off while the daily stress you encounter weighs the see-saw down. The idea is to make your see-saw balance most of the time. It's okay if it teeters because life is not perfectly balanced all the time. Throughout your day your see-saw will weigh heavier on either side depending on what you are doing. The point however is to find enough activities to lighten the heavy side so that the see-saw will work, find its balance, and give you a pleasurable ride. Here's your goal.

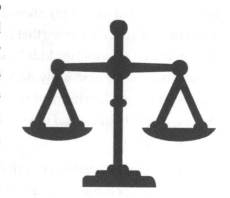

- Take a look at your life and imagine your see-saw. Chances are it's heavy on the responsibility, commitment side and light on the pamper, self care side. Just as the see-saw isn't fun for two kids of unequal size, your see-saw can't be that much fun either. This week commit to working towards balancing the see-saw by adding activities that bring it into balance. Visualize the see-saw lift as you find time for things that bring you joy, passion, and purpose. Add at least one activity and note how as your see-saw comes into balance, you feel less stress, more centered and calm.

In order to live a balanced life, all parts of your life must be in balance. That means more than just getting your eating habits and exercising on track. It also means taking care of your emotional needs, your relationship needs, your spiritual needs, and implementing an effective plan in order to manage and control your stress. Each of these components is crucial for health, fitness, and wellness both inside and out. All are crucial for lifestyle fitness.

If you're still not convinced about the dangers of unmanaged stress, I'll tell you a personal story that may change your mind. Just a few years ago, I spent all of my time, effort, and energy on my growing family, my thriving practice, managing my home, and if there was any extra time, I spent it with my patient husband. Things were running fairly smoothly except I had bursitis in my shoulders and the pain could only be controlled with quarterly shots of cortisone. It seemed that if I weren't battling an upper respiratory infection, I'd catch whatever current virus the kids brought home from school. I had two herniated discs and degenerative disc disease in my neck and upper back that numerous doctors diagnosed as being the cause for my horrific pain (it felt like a knife was piercing through my shoulder blades). At one point, I almost had to stop driving because I could barely turn my head to look over my shoulder.

My skin was breaking out like a teenager, I was losing my hair, gaining weight and I rarely got a good night's sleep. If things weren't uncomfortable enough, I developed such severe arthritis in my feet that I could barely walk! (Every podiatrist I saw attributed such damage to years of running. I was curious as to why some people could run into their eighties and I had to stop before my fortieth birthday!). To ease the pain and continue with my chaotic lifestyle, I had cortisone shots (just like I was receiving in my shoulder) every three months in both feet to reduce the inflammation. Even low heeled shoes caused terrible pain so I almost always wore sneakers or flat shoes.

So there I was a young working mom of four who needed to be "on top of her game" but was living in intense pain with no effective solution. I kept going with the "help" of cortisone shots, caffeine, and sugar. I was a Registered Dietitian who was growing thick in the middle and a Personal Trainer who could hardly walk! Although I ate as well as I could and tried to exercise I was anything but healthy.

At this point I realized that even with a somewhat healthy diet and exercise, living a toxic lifestyle filled with toxic relationships, unmanaged stress, burning the candle at both ends, and trying to be "super mom" was only causing me illness and pain. After countless attempts at pain relief (aspirin, physical therapy, acupuncture), exercise became impossible and foot surgery seemed like the only option left to allow me to resume even moderate activity. Although it would leave me in a cast and crutches for three months I timed the surgery so that while I recovered I would begin my training as a Whole Health Coach so I could better understand how our lifestyles lead us down the path of health and wellness or illness and disease. What I learned was nothing short of fascinating.

Once I completed the necessary courses, I had to write a thesis in order to successfully complete the program requirements. I decided to write about the physical and emotional consequences of chronic stress because I was beginning to notice a strong link between the stress I was under and the physical complications that were popping up as a result. Article after article, study after study, I found myself written on every page! My signs, symptoms, illnesses, and conditions were all so commonly associated with high levels of over-secreted hormones and unmanaged, prolonged chronic stress. I clearly saw how I manifested my stress into a physical and emotional illness or condition and I resolved to erase the damage I'd caused my body and mind.

It was time to change. First I resolved some old emotionally traumatic issues that were consuming my thoughts and actions and keeping my stress level high. Within a short period of time, I began to feel less stress, lighter and freer. Next I began to understand that the majority of physical pain I felt was due to the over-secretion of hormones released as a result of chronic, unmanaged stress. With this new knowledge, some self compassion and a game plan, one by one my symptoms would disappear. My hair began to grow back thicker and healthier, my middle began to regain its pre-stress shape, my skin cleared, I slept better, my back pain ceased, and I eventually was able to walk, run, and get back into my killer heels! I even cancelled surgery for my other foot that was originally scheduled six months after my first surgery. I no longer needed it because I had completely erased the pain through knowledge and understanding! I was back to being the role model I had always hoped to be.

Today I'm happy, fulfilled and completely pain free. I'm stronger than ever, nothing hurts and my body is in its best shape yet. I let go of toxic relationships and emotional anchors that were holding me back and exchanged them for a fresh perspective that served as wings to help me fly. Never underestimate the power of stress and your power to heal yourself through knowledge, compassion, and understanding. Trust me. You have everything you need within you to begin to effectively manage your stress. By doing so, you can enjoy the health, fitness, and wellness benefits that naturally come as a result.

Physical Fitness Program

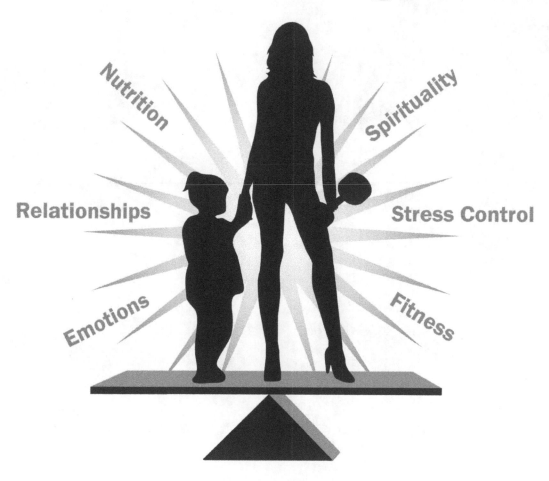

Introduction

It doesn't matter if you are a seasoned athlete or new to exercise. As long as your goal is to improve *your* level of fitness each day and in *any* way, you'll see results. I'll give you two examples.

I used to work with an extremely overweight mom who wanted to become fit enough so she could comfortably walk to her mailbox at the end of her long driveway. She barely had the energy to walk up and down her stairs and was usually out of breath when she opened the door to let me in for our exercise session. We began by placing an egg timer on her children's ping pong table. I set the timer for one minute and she walked "laps" around the table. After one minute, she sat down, caught her breath, and when she was ready, she began her next minute of laps. She progressed minute by minute, day by day. A few weeks after she began, I got a phone call from a woman who was speaking so fast I could barely understand her. Once she slowed down, I realized it was my client. She was calling to tell me that not only did she easily get the newspaper at the foot of her driveway, but saw her neighbor's newspaper across the street. She crossed the street, grabbed her friend's newspaper, rang her doorbell and delivered the exciting "news!"

Another mom I worked with ran track in high school and continued running until breast cancer took away her strength, focus, and vitality. After surgery, chemotherapy, and radiation, she slowly regained the desire to feel fit, healthy, and whole. This strong, courageous mom decided to reclaim her body and mind by signing up for an upcoming 5k breast cancer race to prove to herself she was "back in the game."

We began a walking program that progressed to walking with short bouts of running. The running time became longer, the walking time became shorter and she was eventually back to her old running self. As I inhaled her inspiration with each step she ran, the feeling of empowerment was contagious. If she was willing to run for her cause, I was willing to do it with her. She vowed to finish and I vowed to win. She finished the race and I placed first for my age bracket and third overall. She also finished to flowers, cheers, and the bright, loving smiles of her husband and children. Without the incentive, support, inspiration, and commitment, chances are we may not have tried as hard. It showed us both that there is nothing we can't be, do, or have. We just have to figure out what it is and go get it.

Chapter 1
Why Do *You* Need to Exercise?

W hy do you need to exercise? There are so many positive reasons to incorporate exercise into your life. First of all, exercise reduces your risk for diseases such as heart disease, stroke, diabetes, and obesity. One reason this occurs is because with exercise, you normalize your levels of stress hormones, blood glucose levels, and insulin levels. When these levels are dangerously high or low, they begin to damage your organs, systems, and then impair the way your body functions. Normalizing these levels keeps your body in balance while reducing your risk for disease.

Exercise also helps to reduce your blood pressure, increase your HDL or "good cholesterol," reduces your LDL or "bad cholesterol," clears toxins, increases the quality of your sleep, sharpens your mind, increases energy, and helps to make your heart and lungs stronger and more efficient.

Exercise is also a mood elevator. First of all, when you exercise, you release endorphins, which act as a potent and powerful feel good biochemical within your body. If you've ever heard of a "runner's high," that's the release of these endorphins during aerobic exercise. It feels like this. Imagine being outside on the perfect day, with a clear head, listening to the perfect song and enjoying the feeling of treating your body well. Now imagine you're midway through your workout and you suddenly feel a burst or surge of energy that makes you feel as if you can fly. You are completely "in the zone," you feel weightless and you feel like nothing beats the feeling you're experiencing right at that moment. You may double your speed and not even notice because you just love the feeling and are so completely enjoying the experience. Now those of you who don't exercise may think I'm nothing short of crazy. I can only urge you to give this "high" a try. When you compare it to any chemically induced high, this one is available at any time, free and actually *good* for you!

The other way exercise elevates your mood is by giving you a positive outlet for stress relief, building your confidence by building a more fit body and showing you that you are committed to living a healthier lifestyle. The positive thoughts we experience as a result of these feelings overflow in many areas. Some studies have found that exercise has been an effective tool in the treatment of disorders ranging from anxiety to depression. On a more moderate level, exercise simply makes us feel good. When we feel good, we can better handle the challenges, problems, or difficulties that surface throughout our day. We've taken care of ourselves, which leaves us in a better position to care for others.

Exercise can be used as a form of meditation. The rhythmic movement of your feet during aerobic activity allows you to clear your mind. When your mind is clear, answers you've been struggling to find, options you've been unable to discover and thoughts you've put on the back burner all have an opportunity to be clearly thought about and worked through. I've had many clients tell me that they've come up with their best ideas and solutions to problems while exercising. During one exercise session, one mom planned her husbands entire surprise 40th birthday party, another decided how to remodel her kitchen, another figured out how to respectfully tell her in-laws not to stay at her home for a full two weeks, and another came up with the perfect name for her friend's new business. Talk about multi-tasking!

Finally, when you incorporate exercise into your life, you're not just talking the talk, you're walking the walk. You can tell your children all day long how important it is for them to exercise. But if they see you finding the time to exercise yourself, they may actually believe you enough to try it out for themselves.

Now that you know some of the physical, mental, and emotional reasons to exercise, let's talk about some of the more obvious reasons. Exercise makes your body lean, toned, and strong. Let's face it. Having children can leave your body in less than optimal appearance and you can thank your little ones for the new stretch marks, change in skin tone, sagging, and a few extra pounds that they may have left you with since their arrival. While people will tell you these are some of the "medals of motherhood" I'm going to tell you something else. You don't have to be unhappy with your post-pregnancy body. In fact, you can make your post pregnancy body stronger, sleeker, and sexier than ever before. While you may have a few extra pounds on you, you also may have some new curves. While your skin tone may not be the same, you can certainly tighten up what's lying underneath. The point is it's never too late or too vain to work towards a healthy, fit body.

While exercise is crucial to your post-pregnancy body, here's a note to those of you still building your families. When I was becoming a certified Personal Trainer, I had various opportunities to work with pregnant clients. I felt uncomfortable working with these women without proper training so I earned two certifications in pre/post natal fitness. Besides learning how to train a pregnant woman safely and effectively, I learned two important concepts. The first was that the delivery of your child is an endurance event. You need strength, energy, and stamina to deliver your baby and without it, while always incredible, the entire event will inevitably be more taxing than it needs to be. The second important concept to remember is that the more fit you are during pregnancy, the better you'll handle the pregnancy itself. Swollen ankles, weight gain, difficulty breathing, bending, and moving will be far less difficult to manage if your body is in better shape during your pregnancy term. Of course, consult with your doctor before starting any exercise program. With all of this in mind, it's time for a goal.

WEEKLY GOAL

- What's your motivation to exercise? What does becoming fit offer you? This week, commit to finding your personal reason for beginning or maintaining an exercise routine. The reason can be your health, to improve the way you look, to find an effective outlet for your stress, to show yourself that you are finding time for self-care or finding a way to show yourself you can make a commitment and stick with it. Whatever reason you discover, write it down and review it every day. On days when you don't feel like exercising, reading your words may offer you the incentive to try. Commit to writing down your motivation, review it daily, and note how it inspires you to action.

Chapter 2
Aerobic/Cardiovascular Exercise

What's aerobic exercise? In a nutshell, aerobic exercise is the type of sustained activity where you engage the largest muscles in your body (legs and gluts) for a prolonged period of time. Oxygen is needed to fuel these muscles in order for them to work effectively. Aerobic activity increases the need for oxygen which allows these muscles to perform, helps to flush out toxins within the bloodstream, increases the metabolism, and strengthens the heart and lungs. Aerobic activity also requires sustained energy in the form of calories which are being used to fuel your workout.

Calories stoke the aerobic flame as wood or coal stokes a furnace. Calories expended means pounds lost. I'll give you a simple formula because math is not my specialty. Thirty-five hundred calories equals one pound of fat. If you break that down over the course of one week or seven days, you'll find that in order to lose one pound of fat each week, you need to burn a total of thirty-five hundred calories. So thirty-five hundred calories divided by seven days equals five hundred calories per day to lose one pound of fat each week. There are a few ways you can address this. I guess you can say that's too much and stop right there but that just wouldn't be right. There are two other options. The first is to burn five hundred calories per day with exercise. You burn about one hundred calories every ten minutes while exercising, so a fifty minute aerobic workout may be a reach for some of us. Another option is to burn two hundred and fifty calories and eat two hundred and fifty calories less which equals a total of five hundred calories. Over the course of a week, that's thirty-five hundred calories and one pound of fat. The bottom line here is, when you burn or expend more calories than you take in, you lose weight and when you take in more calories than you burn, you gain weight.

Understanding this formula may also clear up some issues about being discouraged with *only* a one or two pound weight loss each week. Two pounds equal seven thousand calories! That's a tremendous amount of calories to eliminate through less food or more activity. The recommended daily caloric intake for the average woman typically ranges anywhere from fifteen hundred to twenty-two hundred calories each day. So, while you're minimizing your accomplishments, remember that you've either burned or given up a lot of calories in order to lose a pound of fat.

As far as the type of aerobic activity to try, it's a completely personal decision. One mom may love to walk, another may love to run, another may love to dance, hike, use an elliptical machine, Stairmaster, or hit the courts for an hour of singles tennis. It doesn't matter what you do as long as you choose something you enjoy. If you find it torturous you'll hardly look forward to it. If you find it invigorating, rejuvenating and inspiring, mark my words, you'll miss it when you can't do it.

You may also be the type of person who becomes easily bored with routine. If that's the case, mix things up a little bit and discover a few activities you enjoy. Try an organized sport that keeps you moving, or change your pace between high and low intensity while alternating between walking, jogging, or running. You can build a library of fun exercise DVDs or take classes at a nearby health club. Maybe you want to go back to doing something you enjoyed before you had kids like riding a bike or jumping rope. I'll tell you a quick story.

When I was sixteen years old, I had my heart set on my first car but I had no money to buy it. It was a fire engine red Triumph TR7 with a pull down sunroof. (I haven't seen these cars on the road in years). I wanted the car and needed to find a way to earn enough money in order to buy it. I found a job at a nearby, fancy country club where I worked as a pool waitress during the day and a hostess in the main dining room at night. I had no transportation and needed to get to work so I found an easy way to get there. I roller skated! Imagine this picture. I'm wearing a white uniform with my black apron tied around my waist, and I'm roller skating to work in my skates with the hot pink wheels! Anyone who saw me got a great chuckle from the sight but I was in great shape, resourceful, and earned enough money to buy the car I wanted. Besides the pride I felt about my accomplishment, I eventually bought and drove the hottest car in my high school! Recently, I told my kids this story. After they told me how weird I was, I informed them that I'm going to try skating again and anyone who wants to join me is welcome to. I gave my old skates away but found roller derby skates that were similar to the ones I had. Many falls but many laughs later, Disco Debi was back skating along to the same seventies music I'd enjoyed twenty-five years ago! This time, no uniform required. Here's your weekly goal.

WEEKLY GOAL

- How much aerobic activity are you getting in? It doesn't matter where you start as long as you improve from what you did before. If you're currently not exercising and you made an effort to briskly walk for fifteen or twenty minutes, good for you! You've committed to action and you're moving in the right direction. If you're already working out three days per week, find a place to add another day! If you're a seasoned athlete and you're exercising almost everyday, consider cross training to reduce the likelihood of an overuse injury. Try different activities until you find something you enjoy. Some may enjoy group classes while others may prefer to exercise on their own. You can also work out with a friend, Certified Personal Trainer, take your husband, kids, friends, or dog for a walk. Try exercising outside, inside, with a headset, or while watching TV. It's not where you are, it's where you're going. Don't compare yourself to anyone else either. You are unique and require your own specific workout plan. This week, commit to adding one more day by creatively adding it somewhere in your week. That's it, just add one more day.

Chapter 3
Resistance Exercise and Flexibility

Resistance and flexibility training are crucial components to a well rounded exercise program but they're often overlooked. I've seen moms frustrated because they're putting the time in on the treadmill but still don't feel strong and toned. Many of my clients have purposely neglected weight training because they felt they would "get too big." I'll debunk some myths later on but without a resistance training program, you really are shortchanging your body and yourself. I'll explain why.

Have you ever noticed a husband and wife trying to lose weight together? Chances are he's dropping weight like crazy and she's struggling each week to lose a small amount. Besides a number of possible reasons, which we've covered in the Nutritional Fitness Program, one of the greatest differences in why he is losing weight at a quicker pace is that she doesn't have the same amount of muscle mass that he does. Muscle burns calories just by being there while fat burns very little. You see, the fat we have on our bellies, butts and thighs takes up a lot of space, it's very content to stay put and it doesn't need us to fire up our metabolism to keep it in its place. Muscle works very differently. Each pound of muscle burns seventy-five calories per hour just to keep it there! Imagine if your fat or muscle were paying rent to live on your body. Fat lives relatively rent free in a large yet average looking apartment while muscle pays much more but lives in a small yet beautiful penthouse suite.

Muscle also shapes and tones your body, improves your posture, helps prevent and protect your body from injury, maintains your bone mass, and enhances your quality of life. When you feel strong physically, you feel strong and empowered mentally. The strength you feel from building some muscle can also give you the courage necessary to tackle something difficult. I'll give you an example. One of my clients was going through a bitter divorce. She looked forward to "getting out her frustrations" by hitting the weights and sweating from a tough workout. For her, a strong body led to a strong mind. The strength she felt overflowed into her divorce proceedings and she was able to negotiate a mutually agreeable plan for herself, her husband, and their children. Strong body, strong mind.

Muscle also makes you look lean, sleek, and toned. While muscle mass devours calories and helps you lose weight, it also tones a frail, thin body. Have you ever seen a thin woman with no muscle tone? She is jiggling and wiggling much more than a heavier but fit woman. The difference is in the muscle. Imagine a shriveled up balloon. It's lax, slack, and floppy. Now fill it with some air. See how it looks stronger, smoother and sleeker? That's what happens when you add some muscle to your body. It fills out the area giving you a much more toned, sculpted, and fit look.

Now let's talk about how muscle adds to your quality of life. As we age, we lose a significant amount of muscle for each decade we live if we don't make an effort to build or maintain what we have. So here we are, aging, and instead of holding onto our muscle that can help us bend, lift and move more easily, we lose it! Without muscle, basic tasks that we take for granted are much more difficult such as lifting up grocery bags, walking up stairs, getting out of bed, and bending to tie our shoes. If we're not careful to maintain our muscle, we need help to achieve some of these simple tasks that we could easily have prevented.

So now that you know how important muscle is, how do you build some? There are many ways to approach this. You can use household items, dumbbells, resistance bands, weight machines, or just use your own body. For example, if you decide for your resistance program you want to begin by lifting three- to five-pound weights, as long as you're struggling when you're lifting those weighs three to five pounds, you'll see results. I would recommend dumbbells over household items if there is a choice, however, because it puts you in a better "workout mode" and provides and easier grip.

Resistance bands can be a great option as well. They take up very little space and range in tension according to the type you purchase. They also usually come with pictures of how to use the bands, which help direct you to perform the exercises correctly. They're also extremely portable. This makes it easy to take and use right in the hotel room whenever you travel, no excuses.

Weight machines are great in that they provide an added safety feature. When the seat, bar or weight is adjusted according to your frame and fitness level, you are more likely to perform the exercises safely and correctly.

Here's how it works with flexibility training. When you stay flexible, you warm up the muscles so they perform better. The better they are able to perform, the greater the results you will receive. Besides enhancing performance, improving your flexibility helps to prevent muscle soreness after a strenuous workout. The muscles are better prepared and are spared excessive damage as a result of the stretching you've done. Another reason to stay flexible is to help prevent injury. When muscles, joints and ligaments are still and tight, they're much more likely to rip or snap. To understand this easily, imagine a piece of cheese because it's made up of protein just like muscle. When you leave it on the counter it can bend, move easily and it's fairly flexible. If you were to put it in the freezer, it would not be at the temperature necessary to make it flexible and it would easily break in half.

Staying flexible also helps to improve your circulation, mental clarity, and it simply feels good. If you've ever taken a yoga class, you can appreciate the feeling of a warmed up, flexible, and stretched body. If you know anyone who practices yoga simply ask them. They'll probably tell you it makes them feel clear headed, flexible, and relaxed. So, now that you know the benefits of resistance and flexibility training, it's time for a goal.

WEEKLY GOAL

- This week in addition to your cardio plan, stretch before and after your cardio workouts and add one day of resistance training. It doesn't have to be time consuming or complicated. You also may want to look in popular fitness magazines or ask a certified Personal Trainer to set you up with a program that suits your goals and needs. Start with one exercise for your upper body such as a push up (against a wall, modified version on your knees or advanced version), one for your mid section (crunches, reverse curls, or using a stability ball) and one for your lower body (lunges, squats). Start with one set of ten repetitions going slowly and safely and work up to three sets of ten repetitions as you feel ready. Commit to performing these exercises at least one time this week. (You can also sign up for private coaching with me if you need a jump start. Visit www.TheMojoCoach.com and choose the coaching program that feels right to you.

Chapter 4
Your Workout Environment

Your workout environment is critical to your workout success. I've been consulted numerous times about what is the best environment for a great workout, what pieces of equipment are the most important, and where is the best location within the home for a large or compact home gym. Here are some of the tips I've offered to clients that may be of help to you.

The first thing to consider is your financial situation when designing a home gym. You can have a great workout with objects within your home, a great workout tape or DVD and a good pair of running shoes. For example, there are many great DVDs available today where you can choose according to your level of fitness and the type of workout you are looking for. A great resource that can help you choose the appropriate DVD for you can be found by going to www.collagevideo.com. You can even bypass the DVD if you find a program you like on the fitness channel in your area. If neither of these ideas appeal to you, you can go outside and walk, jog, run, or even run up and down your stairs (that's the exact workout you'd get with a stair climber at your local gym). For exercise enthusiasts, jumping rope can give you an intense cardio workout. You'd be amazed at how difficult it is to jump for even one minute! Besides feeling like a kid again, jumping rope is an extremely effective cardio workout but be sure you are physically and mentally prepared for this type of intensity. My good friend Lucie Buissereth is a national jump rope champion and teaches fun jump rope classes for hundreds of moms and kids in the New York area. You can learn more about jump rope cardio by emailing her at www.lucieb.com.

For your resistance training, nothing beats using your own body weight as resistance. For example, let's say you are an average weight woman of one hundred sixty pounds. Sure I could suggest that you hold five pound dumbbells in your hands but how about if you used your own one hundred sixty pounds to press against. You'd be using your own body weight, require no equipment and strengthening every muscle of your body. Examples of resistance exercises requiring no additional weight would be push ups, chair dips, abdominal exercises, squats and lunges for your legs and gluts. Proper form is critical for safety and results so it's best to find someone who can show you these exercises first so you can perform them safely and correctly.

For flexibility training, you can learn a few good stretches and incorporate them into your routine. Nothing needs to be complicated. Concentrate on the muscle you're trying to stretch and you'll know the stretch is working when you feel that muscle gently stretching.

For a moderately priced gym, you can either purchase a gym membership or buy a few items for your home. My experience has been that busy moms often can't find the extra time necessary to go out to a gym. Even if they can, I've worked with many moms who've wanted to get into shape at home just so they feel comfortable enough to join the gym! Clubs are great in that they offer camaraderie, fun classes, and an extra boost of motivation along with babysitting services for your children. But you know yourself best. Results don't happen when you purchase the membership but when you actually use the services. If you can't find enough time to go to the gym, or don't have enough incentive to go there, make it work for you at home. Here are a few ways how.

Depending on your budget, you can purchase a piece of cardio equipment along with resistance bands or dumbbells, a stability ball, and a comfortable mat. If you can purchase one piece of cardio equipment, the first thing to do is try it out before you buy it! Although something may look or sound appealing, unless you try it you can't really know for sure if it's the right piece of equipment for you. Many of my clients have had great success purchasing cardio equipment that was either being sold on eBay, picking something up at a moving sale, or buying the floor model in the fitness store. My experience has shown me that you're better off using a piece of quality equipment at a discount price versus a sub optimal version that is new. If it doesn't feel sturdy, secure and give you the stride or comfort you're looking for, it will only serve as another coat rack within your home. Also, machines become expensive when they are programmed with multiple programs. If you don't intend to use this feature, choose a model that gives you a great workout with fewer bells and whistles.

Now let's talk about your exercise environment. There are a few key points to consider here. First of all, make sure wherever you're working out is spacious enough for your activity, well ventilated and clutter free. Working out in a cramped, messy environment zaps your mental energy, which makes for a more difficult workout. The next tip is, if you have an option of putting your equipment in your basement or on the main floor, go for where there is more light, windows and circulating air. I can't tell you how often I've walked into a clients spacious home only to find the most beautiful and well equipped gym tucked away in a damp, dark basement. The atmosphere is not aesthetically pleasing and the equipment is not as "in your face" so it is rarely used. Just by moving things to a more pleasing environment can stimulate the desire to use what you may already have.

It's also important to make the workout pleasing with some inexpensive additions. You can invest in a ceiling fan or simply place a portable fan nearby. You may be able to stay with your workout longer if you're not terribly overheated. Of course, make sure you have a water bottle nearby and take a few sips before, during and after your workout. You'll need more or less according to the temperature so adjust your intake to suit the weather. If it helps to watch TV to get you through your workout, place the machine so you can watch your favorite show. I had one client who caught up on all of her favorite soap operas during her workout. She loved her soaps but refused to indulge in this treat unless she was on her treadmill. She caught up on all of the latest dilemmas while getting a great workout! Music is also a great motivator to work out with. Play the stereo, listen to your iPod or mp3 player, or you can even download personal training programs, which can be found at www.podfitness.com or www.itrain.com.

This next tip is something that may take some getting used to, but once you do it can be a great way to get through and thoroughly enjoy a tough workout. It involves your favorite book or magazine, a reading rack and "chip clips." I discovered this trick when I was already a Personal Trainer but working towards my Master's degree in Nutrition and becoming a Registered Dietitian. I had to study and I needed to work out so I decided to combine the activities. I took my text book or class notes, placed them on a reading rack (you can purchase these in a fitness store, or your machine may be built to accommodate a book or magazine) and took two small chip clips from my pantry to secure the left and right pages. With the clips in place, the pages didn't move and I was able to study and run at the same time! Before I knew it, my work out was over and I was able to concentrate and retain much more than if I sat down to study. The reading enabled me to not realize how long or hard the run was and the running gave me focus and clarity for my studies! Since that discovery, I've never been on a piece of cardio equipment without a book, book rack, and chip clips. I'm exercising, reading, and the book covers the time display so I don't focus on it.

For those of you who plan to work out at home with small children, this tip is for you. As I mentioned in the introduction, you can use a playpen, indoor swing, exersaucer, or anything else that may keep your children happy and contained. My kids always loved when I wore the baby harness (Baby Bjorn, Snugli brand). They felt close and the rhythmic movement always gave them a great nap! Jogging strollers are also great along with exercise tapes you can do yourself or with your baby.

This last tip involves the clothes you wear when you're working out. The clothes and sneakers you wear need to be appropriate for both the weather and the activity. It's also helpful to wear exercise clothes that motivate you to work out. Ratty T-shirts may get the job done, but when you wear clothes designed for the activity, you may take it more seriously. For example, I used to train a mom who wanted to do her workout in her slippers. She loved the idea that she didn't have to dress up for me and wanted to be comfortable and relaxed. I explained that it's fine to be comfortable but when you're too comfortable, you just don't perform or push yourself the same way. Just by putting on her sneakers, she gave herself a better opportunity both mentally and physically to achieve a better workout. Now, as your Personal Trainer, "drop down and give me thirty pushups!" Only kidding, but it is time for a goal.

WEEKLY GOAL

■ This week, commit to designing your workout environment. Join the health club if you intend to use it or design a gym at home. Your home gym can be as simple or elaborate as your budget allows. Start with the right sneakers for the activity you plan on, and then add on from there. Make your environment conducive to a great workout by providing yourself with the right equipment, essentials and atmosphere that best suits your needs. Move things around, purchase what you need, do whatever you need to in order to get yourself and your space "workout ready."

Chapter 5
How Much, How Often, How Difficult

How much you exercise, how often you exercise, and how difficult your workout needs to be depends on your current fitness level and the results you're hoping to achieve. As I mentioned earlier, as long as you are doing more than you've done before, you're progressing in the right direction, and you're working towards results. That said, you can exercise to feel better, strengthen your heart and lungs, maintain your weight and fitness, or lose weight and reshape your body depending on where you are mentally and physically.

For example, if you're very overweight and don't currently exercise, just beginning a walking program one day this week is more than you've done before. You've set a goal, reached it, feel pride in your accomplishment and want to continue. Feeling better may be the initial incentive that encourages you to begin exercising where as if you are already committed to exercising four days each week, reshaping your body may be what you're looking for.

How often you need to exercise is also based on your needs and goals but also involves your decision to prioritize your workouts. I've heard every excuse there is, and we are incredibly capable of justifying and rationalizing anything we don't want to do. Not having enough time is the most common excuse for not exercising. There are also excuses about the weather, the results you're not seeing quickly enough, your mood, the kids, your fatigue, the full moon, whatever. Each excuse can be countered with an important reason *to* exercise. (Remember a few chapters ago when I asked you to write down your motivation to exercise? It's to counter these excuses that prevent you from fitting it in). My point is if we want to do something badly enough, we find a way to make it happen, period. If exercise isn't a priority at this point, it's just too easy to let it go. Here are a few ways that may help you find time and prioritize your workout.

For years I would write exercise down in my date book just as I would write down any other appointment. I always respected the time and commitment involved with any other appointment so I decided to respect my own exercise time as well. By writing it down, you're making the commitment, planning your day with your workout in mind, honoring yourself, your time, and your needs.

If you can work out in the mornings, it may be your best bet. There are so many things that can come up throughout the day that are tacked on as the day progresses. If exercise was planned for the end of the day, it might just get pushed off the list to ensure the earlier commitments get taken care of. Because there are fewer distractions earlier in the day, you are less likely to be sidetracked by something else. One trick is to start the day by immediately waking up and changing into your exercise clothes. They'll serve as a reminder to get your workout in as soon as you can.

If exercising in the morning isn't possible, make sure you can fit it in by making things easy for yourself. Leave your gym bag packed and in the car, exercise as soon as your children go to bed, dedicate your lunch break to finding time to workout, and make it work however you can. No one said it would be easy, but if you manipulate your schedule enough by rearranging certain things, spending less time on non-essentials, or possibly waking up a little bit earlier you'll find the time you need. Besides finding the time, you're prioritizing your need for a fit body and that sends a strong message to you and those around you that you're committed to a living a healthier lifestyle.

How difficult your workout needs to be depends on a few factors. First of all, you want to challenge yourself but not dread the experience. You want to work out hard enough to see results yet not hurt yourself. Finally you want to find a way to include fitness into your lifestyle. Here, slow and steady wins the race. If you go for that "weekend warrior" approach where a rigorous weekend workout renders you incapable of moving for the rest of the week, chances are it's too aggressive of a strategy to maintain over the long term and you'll give up before feeling or seeing results. With a more gradual approach, you can better incorporate it into your routine, your week and your new healthier lifestyle. How do you know if your routine is difficult enough?

For resistance training, the best way to determine if your program is challenging enough is by checking with your body to see how it feels. If it feels too easy, it probably is and a higher weight or more repetitions may be necessary. A mild soreness twenty-four to forty-eight hours after your workout is a good "reminder" that you've worked out hard enough to achieve results.

For aerobic training, there are two easy tests you can perform to determine how challenging your workout is. The first is called the "talk test" and that's exactly what you do. For example, let's say you're walking with a friend and she says, "How was your weekend?" If you can only manage to squeak out an "okay," chances are you're working too hard. If she asks you the same question and you respond with a fifteen minute summary of the entire weekend, you probably need to pick up the pace. If she asks you the question and you respond with " It was great, we went out, the kids saw some friends, we all had a good time," you're working at the right place and are within your "target heart rate zone," which is the range where you burn the most calories over time. So, when using the "talk test" strive for short sentences.

The other type of test you can perform is called the "rate of perceived exertion." With this test, there is a range from zero to ten, with zero being the least challenging and ten being the most challenging. While working out, rate your exertion. If it's a zero you're sleeping, and if it's a ten you'll need an oxygen mask and an emergency room. Strive for an exertion that you rate to be between six and eight. If you're just starting out, you can stay at a level five but not lower than that if you want to see results. Athletes can push to a nine if they wish, but it's unnecessary unless you're training for a specific event. Since everyone has a different threshold for exertion, determine your own and stay within the guidelines of what feels challenging yet safe for your body.

Now, let's say it's a day you planned on exercising but you're just not feeling it. The thought of exercising is exceptionally unappealing and you'd rather do anything else. Here's where you can try the ten minute rule. With the ten minute rule, you ask yourself to workout for ten minutes and then give yourself permission to reevaluate after that time. If you still hate it after giving it a fair try, stop, try again tomorrow and let it go. What happens very often, however, is that when you just promise yourself ten minutes, you often decide "I'm already doing it, may as well finish" or your muscles may be warmed up after the ten minute mark and you don't mind working out anymore. If you're lucky, you're absorbed with your

TV, music, outdoors, or reading and don't even notice you've passed the ten minute mark. In either case, you're giving yourself a fair shot and permission to give your body what it wants and needs. Here's your goal.

WEEKLY GOAL

- This week, commit to using the "talk test" or "rate of perceived exertion" test to determine how challenging your workout is and adjust accordingly. Schedule your workout time into a date book, write it on your calendar, put on your gym clothes, and commit to overcoming any excuse you may have. If you apply the ten minute rule, use it only once each week. Your goal is to make exercise a priority by moving it up on the ladder of what's important to you. The more of a priority it is, the more likely it is that it will get done. You'll see results and treat yourself to the body you deserve.

Chapter 6
Overtraining, Overuse: When it's Okay to Exercise and When it's Not

S o you're probably thinking, "the more I exercise the better off I am, right?" Well, not entirely. There are times when it's important to ease up, cut back, and not exercise at all. For many moms, getting started with an exercise program is a huge step. Once they're able to begin, they see results, enjoy how they look and feel, and find a way to make exercise a regular part of their routine. While this is great for your health and fitness, there comes a point when we may be overtraining, overusing our muscles, and exercising when we need to take some time off.

Let's start with overtraining. This is when we exercise more than our bodies need or want to. When we exercise excessively, we may need to consider why we're putting in so much time. I've often found that many moms over exercise to compensate for poor eating. For example, the more they overeat, the more they "punish" themselves with extra time on the treadmill. This works against you for a few reasons.

For one, exercise is something that's best when it's enjoyed, especially if it's something you hope to incorporate into your routine in some capacity for life. If we view exercise as a punishment, we've given it a negative connotation. Anything we view negatively we naturally gravitate away from because humans are pleasure seeking. Think negatively about exercise and you'll eventually find a way to avoid it.

The next problem with over exercising as a way to compensate for poor eating habits is that it then becomes another form of purging. Someone who has an eating disorder such as bulimia will ingest large quantities of food then purge the calories by either vomiting or taking laxatives. If you're overeating and then burning those calories by extra time on the treadmill, it becomes just another way to purge those extra calories. The biggest problem that I often see is that because the method of purging is disguised by something normally viewed as healthy (exercise), we justify the behavior and act as if it's normal. Exercising in moderation is normal. It's healthy and beneficial for a variety of reasons. Exercising to make up for unhealthy eating behaviors is not healthy. It's "exercise bulimia" and it eventually catches up with you.

The way over-exercising catches up with you is often in the form of either a suppressed immune system or an overuse injury. Your immune system is what offers you protection against bacterial or viral invasion. It's almost like an internal army protecting its borders. A suppressed immune system is like having that army fast asleep. The enemy can easily get through and invade.

An overuse injury is caused by repetitive action to the same muscles. When we exercise, tiny tears are created in muscles. Within a day or so, they build and repair. This is a normal, healthy process. In an overuse injury, the muscle is broken down from too much use. It doesn't have an opportunity to heal and depending on if the damage is severe enough, surgery is often the only option. Another downside of an overuse injury is the pain it causes and the disruption it can cause to your lifestyle. For example, if you have an overuse injury that leaves you with a torn tendon, muscle, or ligament in your leg you may be unable to drive. An overuse injury in your hand or arm may leave you unable to open a door, twist open a jar, or lift your children. An overuse injury in your back may leave you unable to function at all.

Many moms often wonder: when is it safe to exercise and when is it unsafe when they're feeling under the weather (such as with a cold)? You need to use your best judgment here, but typically, if you're feeling it above the neck (head cold) you may find that some moderate cardiovascular activity actually helps to clear your sinuses. Below the neck (when the infection is in your chest and lungs) means lay low. You're struggling to breathe normally. Exercise will only increase your need for oxygen that you're struggling with already. You also need extra rest when you're sick so take the time to rest and heal.

Now, before you begin any exercise program, check with your doctor first. That said, what do you do if you're exercising and all of a sudden, you feel a pull, strain, or tear? Remember R.I.C.E. That stands for Rest, Ice, Compression and Elevation. Here's your goal.

WEEKLY GOAL

- Are you overtraining? Are you exercising more than one hour each day or organizing your life around your exercise? Are you defensive when you're asked about your exercise habits or neglecting important obligations because you're exercising as a way to burn off calories from a binge? If you are, get to the root of what's going on here and get help if you find you need it. Exercise can be addictive in the best kind of way. It's a great stress reliever, therapeutic, and the benefits are endless when it's used appropriately. When it's used as a form of punishment, purging, or used as a way to avoid something else, it's important to find out why. This week, commit to discovering your reason for overtraining. By cutting back on your exercise, you'll also find a few extra hours you never knew you had!

Chapter 7
Debunking Some Exercise Myths

There are a few myths that have been circulating for a long time and need to be cleared up once and for all. The first one involves the fear of using weights because we don't want to "get bulky." We can never get the bulk we're thinking of without lifting well over our own body weight, putting in at least a few hours each day to strenuously train and having large amounts of testosterone within our bodies. Most women who lift weights using even moderate weight achieve a sleek, sculpted look. Unless you want to look like a world class weight lifter, using moderate weights will not give you that bulky look.

The next myth is that you can lose fat and it can turn into muscle. This is impossible because they are two completely different things. We often believe one turns into the other such as water turning into ice and vice versa. This is incorrect when speaking of muscle and fat. Muscle turning into fat or vice versa is like saying wood can turn into metal; it's just not possible.

Another myth regarding fat and muscle is that fat somehow weighs more than muscle. One pound of fat weighs the same as one pound of muscle. The difference is that muscle is more compact and fat takes up five times the space! Two women can weigh exactly the same amount but be two different sizes depending on what those pounds are made of. If the weight is largely made up of fat she will be larger, but if those pounds are made up of muscle the more muscular woman can wear a size smaller in her clothes.

The next myth involves what is called "spot-reducing." That means that if you have large thighs and commit to hundreds of leg lifts each day you will lose the extra weight on your thighs. This is impossible because fat is systemic just like the blood that travels within your body. Fat can be lost through aerobic activity or through burning calories by building extra muscle. While we can definitely lose fat, we don't decide where we lose it from by performing specific exercises. Those exercises will tone your body and build the muscle you are working, but they will not cause you to lose fat in the area on top of the muscle you are focusing on.

Another myth is the belief that certain people don't sweat. I've heard this one a number of times where moms tell me they don't sweat no matter what type of exercise they do. When you sweat, your body is cooling off from being heated by exercise. If you're not sweating, chances are you're not working out with enough intensity to make you sweat. A simple adjustment to your routine may make all the difference and turn you into a "sweater."

The worst of all possible myths is when you say and believe you can't exercise, become fit, or whatever. By buying into this myth you've sabotaged yourself before you even begin. Your limiting thoughts will prevent you from taking the first steps to become fit and will ensure that you stay convinced that a fit, healthy body is something you can never achieve. Here's where you take that inner critic and tell it to take a hike. You can do anything. Whether you choose to believe it or not, it will surely come true. Here's your goal.

WEEKLY GOAL

- What are some exercise myths you've been buying into that have prevented workout success so far? Have you spent countless hours hoping to lose your belly through crunches alone? Have you resisted resistance training for fear of becoming too bulky? Worst of all, have you told yourself you can't? This week, commit to overcoming every myth and limiting belief that's prevented you from working towards the body you want. Challenge every myth with fact. Tell that inner critic you know best, and remember, you don't have to listen. Most importantly, commit to believing that you can become healthy, fit, happy, and whole. Sure it may take time, energy, and effort, but like I keep saying, nothing really good comes easy.

Chapter 8
Daily Activities, Fidgeting, and the Conservation of Energy

S ure we want to conserve energy, natural resources, money, and whatever else can help us to protect the planet and ourselves. While we've made efforts to become efficient at conserving energy however, we've become proficient when it comes to conserving our own. We buy products designed to make life easier but these products limit the energy we must spend. Electric garage door openers, television remotes, electric can-openers, dishwashers, drive through windows, and baby monitors enable us to stay put so we don't have to get up and move. If you used to hand deliver a note or message to someone at another desk at work, you can easily email them. If you gamble, you'll notice how you don't even have to pull the lever on a slot machine any more!

So many products and services make things simpler and easier yet all of this energy conservation is making us bigger than ever. In a nutshell, the more "efficient" our world becomes, the less "efficient" our bodies become at burning calories.

Take a minute to think of someone who's naturally thin. Not someone who lives from one diet to the next or rarely eats a meal but someone who maintains their weight with seemingly relative ease. One thing you may notice is that they rarely conserve energy. When they need something, they'll get up to get it versus asking you to pass it to them. When they want to get somewhere, they'll move at a quick pace versus strolling along. When they have free time, they'll often choose an activity that requires movement such as gardening versus a more sedentary activity such as watching TV. Naturally thin people are often not as physically "efficient" as overweight people. They won't wait until things pile up before taking them upstairs, wait for the elevator when the stairs are right there, or wait for the closest parking spot to prevent a longer walk. They don't think about the extra movement, they just do it.

Naturally thin people may also be found fidgeting. Studies have found that fidgeters burn much more than their more sedentary contemporaries. Their bodies are constantly moving whether doodling, rocking while waiting on a line or pacing while on the phone. Movement expends energy (calories) and although it may not look like much, this energy adds up over the course of the day.

If there's no naturally thin adult you know, take a look at your kids. If they need to get somewhere, they don't walk in order to get to where they want to go, they run, jump, skip, hop, bounce, or glide! If you're exhausted following a young child around all day it's because they're constantly moving. The reason you want to hold their hand half the time when you're in a busy area is because they move so fast if you don't hold on to them, they'll quickly run ahead! There's no conservation of energy with them, just bursts of movement and action. So, if you're sedentary, physically "efficient" or you're an "energy conservationist," this goal's for you.

WEEKLY GOAL

■ This week, decide how you've been conserving your energy in order to "make life easier." While it may make things easier, the extra energy you'll gain from additional movement will make you feel healthier and stronger. Once you've decided how you've been conserving your energy, decide on two ways to move more. Commit to pacing versus sitting while on the phone. Purposely park further away and walk the distance or take the stairs instead of the elevator EVERY time. Commit to adding more daily activity by adding two ways you'll be LESS energy efficient!

Chapter 9
Scales, Tape Measure, Fat Testing, and Loose Pants

How do you recognize weight loss success? This is once again a personal decision. Some measure success by the pounds on the scale. (Remember, from the Nutritional Fitness Program section, pounds lost on the scale can mean fat, water, muscle, or all three). Some moms measure their success by using a tape measure and recording measurements periodically. Others choose to be professionally tested using skin calipers or more extreme measures like hydrostatic weighing where you're weighed in a special chamber in a pool of water. Still others judge weight loss and fitness by the way their clothes fit or the compliments they receive.

There are positives and negatives you'll find with each, so it's important to understand them all in order to determine what works best for you. Let's start with the scale. Sure it can be motivating when the needle moves to the left but what about if you're working out and building muscle? Now you're adding pounds but changing the composition of your body and while you may look better, a scale that refuses to budge may bring you unnecessary frustration. Also, often during weight loss, we reach a plateau. Our bodies aren't computers and may not lose weight with exact precision. You may not show a weight loss for a few weeks and then show a fairly dramatic weight loss all of a sudden. If you go by the numbers on the scale alone, you may become discouraged.

The next method many moms choose is measuring themselves with a tape measure. This can be very motivating or discouraging depending on who's doing the measuring and the results you get. I've worked with moms who've been so aggravated with their bodies that the thought of taking measurements is nothing short of terrifying. Although it may serve as an effective benchmark, many moms find it a discouraging way to begin their program. For them, it's more damaging initially than it's worth in order to see their progress later on. For some moms, using a tape measure works well. If this works for you a good rule of thumb is to measure the same upper arm, upper thigh, waist, hip, and bust. It's important to measure the same time and same day from month to month (to be able to have a chance to see progress and avoid measuring excess water retention from PMS, etc.). Write the numbers down, compare from month to month and enjoy your success!

For some moms, the best way to judge weight loss and fitness success is by noting how they fit and feel in their clothes. To be more specific, I always encourage moms to find one particular pair of pants that they're trying to get back into. It doesn't matter if you can't even get them past your knees. From week to week (trying them on at the same time and day from one week to the next) try the pants on and notice how they fit. If they couldn't go past your knees and this week they do, that's progress! If they're over your knees and start creeping up your thighs, good for you! This can be a very private and personal tool you choose to note your progress. If you choose not to be so private about it, it's great to share this success with me! Make sure to use your special access link to let me know about your victory at www.TheMojoCoach.com/contact.php

You may find yourself in dangerous territory if you judge weight loss success according to the compliments you receive. Some people may not notice because they are preoccupied with other thoughts and you may misinterpret that into thinking that your weight loss doesn't show. Others may neglect to tell you because they may feel that by commenting, they noticed you were heavier before, so to spare potentially hurting you, they choose to avoid it altogether. Others may feel uncomfortable, jealous, or envious of your weight loss success. So the best person to try to impress is you. You know your body best and you know how it changes through hard work. It's best to impress yourself and reward yourself for all your effort instead of waiting, hoping, or expecting someone else to do it for you. Once again, if you are looking for a little pat on the back, let *me* share in your well deserved success! Here's your goal.

WEEKLY GOAL

- How do you measure your changing body? It's important to find a way to recognize your achievement in a way that is motivating and encourages you to continue. This week, commit to a way to determine weight loss and fitness success. Make sure it's one way, stick to it, and don't vary between many methods. This will be your personal measurement tool that will serve as a way to mark your success. The idea is to see the success and feel proud, inspired, and happy with your results. This week, find a way that works for you, commit to it and use it from week to week to measure results.

When we incorporate exercise into our lives, we send a powerful message to ourselves and others that we are dedicated, committed, strong, vital, empowered, healthy and whole. Besides enhancing us physically, we've enhanced ourselves mentally, emotionally and spiritually as well. We've prioritized fitness in order to receive the many benefits it brings. We've found a healthy, positive outlet to deal with the stressors of our day as opposed to something either destructive or harmful. We've also shown ourselves that we deserve some self care in the form of a body that looks and feels good from the inside-out. A strong body helps build a strong mind and is a crucial component when building a healthy lifestyle. By incorporating a realistic fitness program into your routine, you are giving yourself an opportunity to embrace life with the help of your outer and inner newfound strength. Good luck!

Emotional
Fitness Program

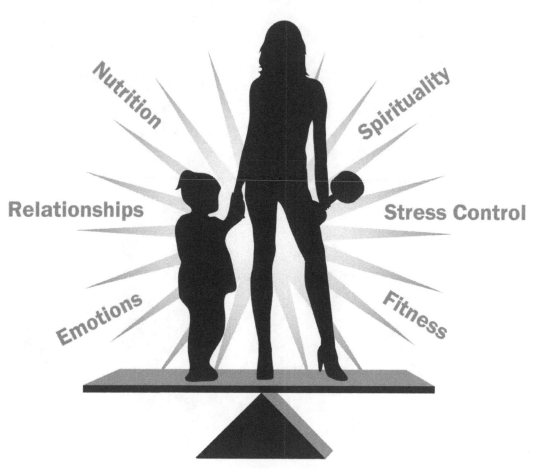

Introduction

When we made the decision to become moms, we had certain expectations about how motherhood "should" be. We may have thought it would be filled with precious moments, laughter, and nothing but special times, but we were slapped instead with the reality of dirty diapers, temper tantrums, runny noses, endless carpools, sleepless nights, and hours of second-guessing every decision involving our precious babies. This is the crucial moment when many moms blame themselves and feel they must have done something wrong instead of frankly admitting that motherhood isn't always perfect. We think we must be bad moms if we don't love the drudgery of some daily tasks and fear it is a poor reflection on ourselves if we even feel guilty, let alone admit it to anyone. No one is saying you don't love your children, but why is it so difficult to admit that we may not like wiping dirty bottoms all day? Why do we feel inadequate if we don't devote every waking moment to our child's endless needs? Why are we riddled with guilt if we fight to maintain any form of self while raising little ones?

One of the answers lies in the fact that we look at other moms to see how well they seem to do it all. Seeing them never lose patience and always staying calm no matter what their children may be doing leaves us feeling unhappy with our own inability to do the same. First of all, any mom who seems to be sailing through motherhood effortlessly either has "mother's amnesia" or is just plain lying. She's also showing you the side of herself that she wants you to see. We have an enormous amount of pressure, stress, and anxiety today because mothers are expected to "do it all" and do it all well. We don't help our case when we try to keep up with these unrealistic expectations. So often we fall short because we are simply human. While being a mom may be the most important job you'll ever have, there is more to you than just that. You have needs, wants, hopes, wishes, desires, and dreams that can't always be put on the back burner just because your child's ideas about what he or she needs conflict with your own. Until you decide that your happiness, wellness, and health matter too, you will feel the intense pressure, continual disappointment, endless frustration, and never-ending discouragement that comes from attempting to live up to these unrealistic expectations that you've bought into.

This Emotional Fitness Program is crucial to your wellness. It's about taking some pressure off and realizing that as long as you do the best you can, you're doing right by your kids and yourself. It's also about realizing that losing it every once in a while, not getting it together from time to time, and not staying up all night to make the perfect cupcakes for preschool is both normal and healthy. We're not Stepford Wives raising Stepford children. We're mere mortals doing the best we can. Besides, wouldn't you want your kids to see that it's okay to make mistakes, show emotion, and learn how to figure out some things for themselves? It's time to get real, moms, and I'm going to make you feel better by telling you a little story about your fearless leader.

I had three children under six years old and I was in my ninth month of pregnancy with my fourth. We'd outgrown our house and decided to rebuild it because we loved our location and neighborhood. We placed a fourteen-by-fifty-two-foot, two-bedroom trailer on our front lawn so we could keep tabs on the project and stay nearby. I had a full-time housekeeper at the time because I was leaving at 4:30 a.m. to train clients by 5:00 a.m. in their homes. My housekeeper had her own bedroom, my two older children (who were five and six at the time) slept in the living room, and my eighteen-month-old toddler was in our bedroom in a toddler bed at the foot of our bed (my fourth child also slept in that room with us after he was born). We only had one dog at the time, and he lived wherever he managed to find space.

When I was finished working, I would drag the kids with me (because I felt guilty leaving them home), and we'd spend our free time choosing tile, handles, doorknobs, and paint chips for our new home. Although my head was spinning from all of the choices available and my lack of decorating ability, I tried to convince them that this was great fun while they fought in the stroller or shopping cart.

In the trailer, the walls were so thin that raindrops sounded like metal pellets banging on the roof. The linoleum tile in the kitchen would puff up like a parachute whenever the heat was on, the bathroom was the size of an airplane bathroom, and all of us always seemed to have to use it at the same time. One day, the power went out, leaving us without hot water. I had to bathe the children and myself, and the only way to get hot water was by running it through the coffee pot (somehow that outlet worked), quickly mix it with water in the tub, and repeat as many times as necessary. After my son was bathed, he skateboarded back and forth across the kitchen floor to unpuff it, and the other kids were crying because my toddler had poured syrup on my other daughter's homework. I lost it. Not just a little but in a way that made me wonder if I was a crazy person. Just then, my husband came in and asked, "Why are the workmen still here? I thought they would have left for the day by now." I looked out the window and to my horror, the entire construction crew had heard every crazy word and quickly turned their heads when they saw my face.

Around that same time, I took the kids to buy Halloween costumes. Now, before I had kids, I would be mortified if I ever saw a mom losing patience with her kids. I swore I'd never be one of "those moms," but then again, I had never shopped for "the perfect costume" with three tired, indecisive kids.

After changing their minds about a thousand times, the children seemed happy with their final decisions. We had spent almost an hour in the store already with way too many people fighting for the same costumes and attention from the sales staff. I asked the kids repeatedly before we got to the checkout counter, "Are you sure this is the one you want? Once we wait on this long line and buy it, that's it." Three little faces finally nodded in agreement, so I walked up to the counter, my kids and my huge pregnant belly in tow.

There were about ten other groups of moms and kids ahead of us and as usual, one of my kids needed to find a bathroom immediately. Spot saved and bathroom found, we got back in line. Just as it was our turn, my son burst into tears because he chose the wrong color Power Ranger costume. Maybe another mom would have quietly calmed her child, left the line, and spent another hour finding the right color, but not this mom. I lost it right there in Party City, quickly paid for "the wrong costume," and stormed out. I was the perfect witch, and I didn't even need a costume to prove it. Did I feel humiliated and mortified by my outburst? Of course I did. Did I apologize later to my son for yelling at him? Yes. Did I exchange the costume the next day for the right one? Yes. While I dreaded seeing the same sales staff who may have witnessed "the event" the night before, I came to the conclusion that my defini-tion of success needed to be redefined, and doing the best I could at the time became a new model of behavior worth shooting for. I also realized that those young kids who worked at the store probably felt the same way about me that I felt about those other pressure-cooked moms I had seen so many years ago. I reaffirmed my vow never to judge another—especially a mom.

Chapter 1
Your Thoughts

The results of one survey showed that 70 percent of moms found motherhood extremely stressful. Over 30 percent of moms with young children were depressed, and 95 percent of moms experienced some form of guilt about parenting. Clearly, we're not always happy, but we sometimes fail to challenge the idea that we can be more positive, happy, and fulfilled if we reprogram our thinking and alter our perspectives. Many of the beliefs you currently have hold you back and hold you down. We'll dismantle each one before leaving this section. But before we go further, it's important to understand that every thought brings about a biochemical response that is interpreted as either positive or negative.

Positive thoughts make us feel happy, excited, and joyful. Negative thoughts make us feel unhappy, uncomfortable, angry, hopeless, and helpless. As humans, we're geared toward survival, and these positive or negative emotions provide an accurate measure of how we perceive our safety and security. When we feel safe and unthreatened, we can be relaxed, calm, and happy—we feel positive emotions. When we feel unsafe or perceive a threat, we can be anxious, afraid, and unhappy—we feel negative emotions. We control these thoughts because they are based on our interpretation of the messages we see. It's important to understand that these thoughts can be changed, and you're the only one who can change them.

The way it works is that we experience something and attach a thought to the event derived from our beliefs and prior conditioning that includes attitude, cultural upbringing, personality, or values. That thought is determined by our basic need for safety and drive for survival. A feeling is produced in response to how we interpreted that thought, based on our beliefs and prior conditioning, and then the brain produces a biochemical response that results in a positive or negative emotion. If you perceive the event as a threat to your survival, you will experience a negative emotion, and if you don't perceive a threat, you'll experience a positive emotion. That's why your reality is unique to you. It is based on your unique interpretation of the events around you and how you felt and behaved as a result of that interpretation.

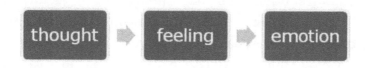

For example, let's say you've been conditioned to believe that having fun means you're not being a responsible adult, and by acting silly, you're setting a poor example to those around you. If you bought into this belief and made it your own, whenever you may have wanted to act silly, you quickly caught yourself and prevented the silly behavior. In short, you've decided that having fun is bad, and you feel a negative emotion when you want to have fun. In this instance, your security was threatened because you felt you'd lose your family's or friend's approval by acting differently from them. So, you maintained your serious behavior to spare yourself from feeling isolated.

But let's say your friend down the block was raised to believe that having fun was what life's all about and believed that depriving herself of fun was like depriving herself of oxygen. Your friend is conditioned to have fun and may catch herself when she's taking herself too seriously. To her, fun is good, and it brings about a positive emotion. Her safety with those around her was never threatened when acting that way, leaving her no need to curb the behavior. Because our brain remembers experiences that resulted in strong emotions, it uses that information to assume the same emotional reaction whenever we encounter the same or a similar event.

Imagine the day after a snowstorm. If you pave a path with your footprints and use that path day after day, the path becomes easy to walk on. Little thought is required to get to where you need to go, so you continue to walk over well-worn footprints. If you were to begin to veer off the paved path, however, your journey may be more challenging. You would need to make new footprints. But over time, if you continued to walk in these new footprints, you would begin a new path that would soon become as worn as the first. That's what happens with our thoughts and our perceptions of certain events. We think and react the same way because of how we've been conditioned. We dare not veer off track even if the thoughts drive us to feel helpless, hopeless, anxious, frustrated, and fearful. We're walking on a well-worn path that doesn't serve us well even though we'd benefit greatly by veering off the path and making the effort to pave a new way. When you reprogram your thoughts, you're making a conscious decision to veer off the path you've been taking by questioning your automatic responses. By doing so, you might just discover something more interesting and beautiful as a result. If you question your response whenever you want to have fun and decide to take that chance and change your thinking, you can pave a new path to react to silliness the same way your friend did. Once you try it out, you realize that your security isn't threatened, that it feels great to loosen up and have fun, and you see the benefit in creating a new path. With effort, you can stop replaying the tape in your head that may be filled with negativity, guilt, self-doubt and defeat…and change it to something that suits you better.

I'll give you another example of a negatively conditioned belief. My youngest son doesn't like my cooking. No matter what I prepare, he's conditioned his thoughts to assume that he won't like whatever I make. One evening, the kids were setting the table and my son asked in one sentence without even a pause, "Mom, what are you making *I don't like that!*" I never even had a chance to tell him what I was making! He was so conditioned to think that he wouldn't like the meal that he had a meltdown from the question itself!

Do you have an endless loop of limiting beliefs that are hurting your growth, development, learning, and fun? Could you benefit from a little bit of reprogramming? If so, this goal's for you.

WEEKLY GOAL

- This week, become aware of any time you respond to a limiting conditioned belief either out loud or to yourself, and determine what is at the basis of your belief. If you say, "I could never do that"; "good moms never lose their tempers or patience"; "I'm such a bad mom," counter the limiting belief with a positive, such as "I could do it if I learned how"; "everyone loses their temper or patience sometimes"; "I'm doing okay." Try out the new phrase as you test the waters to find a more pleasing belief. Repeat the positive belief often enough so that it eventually sticks. Have you ever heard the term, "Fake it till you make it?" Even if you don't believe it yet, when you continue to rephrase negative beliefs into positive ones, you reprogram your thoughts, create a new internal tape, and learn to think, feel, and react in a more positive, empowering way. This week, commit to reprogramming those dangerous, damaging thoughts. Remember, you're the only one who has the ability to change them.

Chapter 2
Accept It, Change It, Forget It

Are you the type of mom who is constantly speaking negatively about yourself, putting yourself down, and complaining about your faults? If your opinion of yourself is that you're not good enough, worthy, or lovable enough, what's the message you're sending to others? How about if you're criticizing your body, your hair, your clothes, or your coping skills? I bet if your friend were putting herself down, you'd stop her immediately and tell her how worthy, beautiful, and lovable she is. If your child suffered from a low self-esteem or poor self-image, you'd spend every free second reassuring him and trying to build him up. So here's the question. Why are we so good to others yet so unforgiving with ourselves?

First of all, it's okay to have limitations. We all have quirks, faults, idiosyncrasies, and limitations. No one is great at everything and that's okay. It makes life more interesting to see in others qualities that are unique and special to them. But when we focus on our faults, they overshadow our strengths and sabotage our self-esteem. They also prevent us from discovering hidden talents, untapped skills, and higher aspirations because we've chosen to spend our energy in a negative, stagnant place. Now, if we have certain limitations and we really have no interest or desire in improving them, why not take the pressure and focus off, then make the decision to accept that limitation lovingly and let it go?

For example, I'm not a gourmet cook. While I make some great meals and desserts, devoting more time to learn how to prepare elegant, gourmet meals on a full time basis is just not on my list of priorities right now. Instead of struggling with the idea that I'm not a world famous chef, putting excess pressure and stress on myself, I accept the limitation and let it go. At this point being frustrated or upset about my limitation would be unfair because I haven't done much to work towards that goal. If I put my mind to becoming a great gourmet chef however, I would eventually learn and wouldn't need to accept the limitation. So now imagine me upset, frustrated, and angry with the fact that I wasn't a gourmet chef. Wouldn't it sound silly? If I haven't invested the time, it's in my best interest to accept my limitation and let it go. Once time, energy, and effort were invested and if at that point I still wasn't a great chef, I could either find another way to change in order to learn the skill, or accept it and let it go.

Now think of how many times you may feel upset about things that you may have been able to control, didn't put forth your best effort yet were unhappy with the results you received. For example, I had a client who constantly focused on her overweight body. She put herself down, complained about how much she disliked the way she looked, and felt constantly miserable with herself. To make herself feel better, she overate and over-spent. While she was great when we were together, her daily binges prevented weight loss and her poor self-image prevented the search to find another alternative. The first step was our weekly appointment, but without taking further steps, weight loss success was unlikely. Discouraged with herself, she refused to acknowledge any strength in any other aspect of her personality because all she saw was weakness and failure when she looked in the mirror.

What would have happened if instead of focusing on her body, which she disliked, she focused on one of her strengths? She was one of the most creative people I'd ever known. She had enormous creative and artistic talent. Instead of focusing on her weakness, by focusing on her strength she would have been in a better position to start feeling better about her accomplishments as opposed to feeling frustrated by her faults. She would have seen that she had qualities worth admiring in herself which may have lead to a place of greater purpose or fulfillment. Maybe she could have become a decorator, artist, or taken some courses to find out which aspect of art proved the most interesting. Once pursuing various options, maybe she would have become excited about a new hobby, interest, or possible career choice which would have lead to feeling more satisfied as she enjoyed her newly found skill. Instead of going this route however, she chose to remain committed to complaining about her body and herself. This is how we limit ourselves.

If you find that you're complaining about something, it's because you think there can be a better way. That means if you're complaining about the size of your thighs, the messiness in your home, or your lack of effective coping skills, it's because you feel things can be another way, and with effort, it can be changed to a way that better suits you. You don't find many people complaining about the fact that we have day or night. It's something we need to accept, it's not changing, and it does no good to fight or question it. We simply adjust our lifestyles to accommodate to the fact that we have certain hours of daylight and certain hours of darkness. Because it would be futile to be upset about this fact, we accept it and let it go. This same theory can easily be applied to either changing what you don't like or accepting yourself and letting it go. When you complain, use it as an important message that if you're complaining about something, deep down you know it can be changed. If you choose not to change it, make the decision to end the complaints, accept things and let it go.

When you want something enough, you find a way to pursue your goal until it's achieved. Think back to any skill you currently have. At one point you didn't possess the skill, but with effort, you achieved that goal. If it wasn't important to you, it may have been easy to accept the limitation and let it go, but if you deemed it important enough, you have that skill today. It boils down to figuring out what you want and finding a way to make it happen. If you don't want it badly enough, accept the limitation and let it go. Everything is possible but you must change your mindset first. Most often, your negative thoughts are your greatest obstacle to overcome.

WEEKLY GOAL

- What are you complaining about that you can either change or accept and let it go? It's just not fair to yourself and others when you focus on your weaknesses instead of your strengths. You have incredible qualities that are being covered by all the negative qualities you choose to share. This week, commit to recognizing complaints as a call to action. For example, no complaining about your schedule if you over commit, no complaining about your body if you're overeating, no complaining about your husband if you've neglected to tell him your needs, no complaining about the dog if you brought it into your home. Make a list of everything you complain about then find a way to fix it or accept the limitation and let it go.

Chapter 3
How Your Thoughts Create Disease (Dis-ease)

Negative thoughts exhaust and weaken the body as opposed to positive thoughts which rejuvenate and refresh. Every thought we have results in a biochemical response that provides us with either positive or negative emotion. Every cell we have is capable of receiving and storing the chemical information from these emotions so when we constantly flood ourselves with negative emotion, we change our cellular makeup with the flood of biochemicals being secreted into our cells. Because certain sites are more vulnerable to this type of alteration, when changes are severe enough, these become the areas where illness and disease often originate.

An example of how negativity can influence disease can be seen in the next study. The study was conducted because researchers noticed that the majority of heart attacks occurred on the same day at around the same time. The day was Monday, and the time was between eight and nine o'clock in the morning. It became known as "parking lot syndrome" because these attacks frequently occurred when arriving to work on a Monday morning. The study found that those who suffered from "parking lot syndrome" had two similar characteristics. The first was job dissatisfaction and unhappiness, and the second was a lack of joy. It wasn't the job necessarily but how that person felt about their position within the company. Maybe they felt frustration about their role within the company, believing they should have a higher salary, better boss, or more responsibility. They may have felt anxious about their job security, workload, or demands placed upon them. Finally, it's likely they felt hopeless or helpless about their ability to change their work situation or environment.

The second characteristic these people shared was a lack of joy. Their work along with their responsibilities and commitments consumed their time and their thoughts leaving them no time, effort or energy to pursue anything positive. Their lives were stressful; they had no healthy outlets to deal with their stress and suffered mentally and physically as a result. This study showed how a threat to safety, security, and survival (the person's expendability and position within the company) resulted in negative emotions leading to disease.

While negativity can contribute to disease, a positive attitude can play an important role in improving conditions, alleviating symptoms, and encouraging wellness. A study that showed how important a positive attitude was in improving health was conducted using breast cancer patients. In this study, patients were divided into four groups based on their attitudes, beliefs, and personalities. The first group had a fighting spirit. They were determined to fight their disease and put their cancer into remission. The second group was in denial. They pushed their fears and anxiety "under the rug" because it was too difficult to face. The third and fourth groups felt more pessimistic, hopeless, helpless, and powerless.

The study found that 80 percent of those with a fighting spirit put their cancer in remission for over ten years. A little over 50 percent of those from the denial group were cancer free for over ten years and only 20–30 percent of those from the hopeless, powerless groups were alive after the ten year mark. What this study and others clearly show is how our attitudes predispose us to disease. We can be consumed and overwhelmed or find healthy, appropriate ways to deal with situations as they arise.

When we have effective coping skills and view life from a more positive perspective, we feel emotionally strong. This view is more in line with the perspective of an optimist. An optimist isn't someone who's in denial; instead they've developed strategies to handle difficult situations as they arise. They aren't as likely to take things personally and feel less hurt, insulted, and stressed as a result. Instead of looking at something as hopeless or negative, they view it as an opportunity for learning and growth. They understand that failing is an important aspect of learning and use failed attempts as stepping stones to greater success. They experience pain but use it as a means of comparison to appreciate joy.

A pessimist's view comes from a more cynical perspective. They expect negative results and an unfortunate outcome. When something negative occurs, it simply confirms what the pessimist expected all along. The pessimist doesn't understand that the life they are living is due to the reactions they've created from the thoughts they've felt. They dwell on the negative, never considering that they have the personal power to change the results they see. They are reactive versus proactive and fail to control their lives, leaving their lives controlling them.

Not long ago, I conducted my own informal study. One of my favorite morning shows is *The Today Show* and I watch it nearly every morning. One of the anchors, Willard Scott has a segment where he shares birthday wishes for people over one hundred years old. I wanted to see if there was any correlation between longevity and certain characteristics so I noted what hobbies, interests, and personality traits were common among the people celebrating this milestone. Time after time it became evident that these people didn't enjoy longevity due to luck but because of attitude! Many worked well into their later years, enjoyed hobbies, and had meaningful relationships. They understood the importance of a positive attitude and lived each day with that thought in mind. That's not to say they didn't have their share of adversity or hardship, they just found a way to see the light at the end of the tunnel. Will you be an optimist by your one hundredth birthday? Here's your goal.

WEEKLY GOAL

- Are you an optimist or a pessimist? Now that you know how your attitude can play such a crucial role in your health and wellness, it's time to be more optimistic for your health's sake (besides having more fun). This week, catch yourself whenever you have a cynical or pessimistic thought. Evaluate it to see if it's justified. If it is, feel the feeling without any judgment, and determine a more optimistic response. No one is saying to disregard your feelings, simply put them in perspective using a more optimistic frame of mind. If it seems impossible, that's your first clue that pessimistic responses are holding you back from changing. This week, commit to taking steps to become more optimistic. Who knows, maybe you'll be featured as someone celebrating a milestone birthday one day.

Chapter 4
Your Inner Guide Versus
Your Inner Bully

Y ou have two internal voices that vie for your attention. One is that quiet voice that gently prods you to follow your instincts, trust your intuition, and "go with your gut." This voice speaks to you through your senses. Maybe you feel a shiver going up your spine, the hair on the back of your neck stand up, goose bumps appear on your arms, or you may just get an unexplainable "feeling" to do or say something. Some explain it as a feeling where they "just know." Learning to strengthen and trust this voice is in our best interest as it isn't clouded or affected by any interference such as ego, judgment, insecurity, fear or self-doubt. It's the voice that knows you best, knows what's best for you and will guide you appropriately if you would only pay attention.

The other voice that struggles for your attention is much louder, more brazen, nastier, crankier, more judgmental, cynical, and critical. That's your inner bully that speaks negatively, fails to give you credit where credit's due, takes over where someone else's negative comments left off, keeps you feeling like a misbehaved child, doesn't want to be challenged, and wants to keep you feeling insecure and unhappy. Unfortunately, this voice plays much louder and more consistently, so it gets stronger and stronger over time. It easily speaks over the gentle speaking inner guide and commands your full attention. By listening, you are kept in your place and left to believe that a better life is out of your reach. This is the way your inner bully continues to be alive and well within you. As long as you'll listen, it will speak to keep you down and out of the game. So here's a thought. How about talking back!

First of all, there's nothing wrong with you. You are capable and fine. You are just being affected by all of the perfection and extreme mothering you see and hear around you, comparing yourself to these ideals and finding yourself coming up short because you are listening to that inner critic who is constantly criticizing, berating, labeling, judging, and telling you how unfit and inadequate you are. Just because that inner critic is saying those things, why do we need to listen? Those negative thoughts have been limiting us for years. They are limiting beliefs that keep us unfulfilled, unsatisfied, and unhappy. They play in an endless loop and keep any higher aspirations at bay. We all come with flaws and faults, why focus on yours?

If you knew that only one song would be played on the radio all day and you didn't like the song, wouldn't you change the station if you could? The same idea can be applied here. The message being conveyed may not feel good, may not be positive and may inhibit your growth, learning and development. Knowing that, why would you continue to listen?

You have a few choices here. One option is to tune it out just as your children tune you out when you're barking orders at them. It's nothing personal; they just don't want to hear it and choose not to listen. Another suggestion is to imagine that inner bully living in your head with a name, a face, and a personality. Name it some ugly name and imagine it looks like a character from a movie or someone you didn't like from your past. Give it a real identity. Now imagine talking back to that character or person and telling it exactly how you feel. When your inner bully is telling you that you're untalented, incapable, and unlikely to change, stand up for yourself and talk back! No one or no thing can bully you without your approval. As Eleanor Roosevelt said, "No one makes you feel inadequate without your consent." Your inner bully is alive and well as long as you give it power. When your "bully" loses its power, it has lost its purpose and retreats. This week, it's time to send it packing. Here's your goal.

WEEKLY GOAL

- Are you listening to your inner guide or your inner bully? Chances are your inner bully is running the show. This week, commit to strengthening your inner guide by trusting your intuition, going with your gut, and following a feeling. While the messages may be faint, just like a muscle it strengthens with use. At the same time, weaken the power of your inner bully by choosing to ignore it or challenge it by talking back. Remember, that bully is only around because you've given it a place to stay. Weaken its power and watch it slink away.

Chapter 5
Self-Medicating Behaviors

W hen we have a negative or unresolved feeling or issue, it's natural to want to alleviate the pain, frustration, anger, or anguish. We want to feel better, safer, more relaxed, or calmer. Maybe we don't want to feel anything and we just want to numb ourselves from the stress, pressure, and strain that we're feeling. While the goal is to feel better, understanding what we do is a valuable tool to finding out what it is that we truly need. Without this understanding, all we can do is self-medicate, writing our own prescription for pain relief.

Self-medicating behaviors are behaviors used with the intention of making us feel better. Just as you may take aspirin to alleviate a headache, self-medicating behaviors are the behaviors we've taught ourselves to bring us serenity and calm. These behaviors can be overeating, taking drugs, smoking cigarettes, drinking alcohol, overspending, overworking, and even over-exercising. When we partake in any of these behaviors, we are trying to make ourselves feel better by using the body's biochemicals such as serotonin, dopamine, or endorphins to flood ourselves with a better feeling than what we had before.

Let's take overeating for example. During a carbohydrate binge, we flood ourselves with a surge of serotonin, the body's feel-good chemical. When we consider why the binge began, it can always be traced back to a trigger that presented a threat to a person's security, safety, or survival. While the binge certainly doesn't solve the problem, we're medicating ourselves with serotonin to feel better. Although temporary and destructive, it's often the medication of choice because we don't need a prescription, it's always available and no one is judged because they purchase food (we all need to eat, right?).

Any one of these excessive behaviors stems from a need to either feel safer, more comfortable or more relaxed. That's why berating yourself for self medicating is destructive to your well-being and discourages changing the behavior. You're only creating more of a need to feel better and self-medicating is the only way you know how to accomplish this. By understanding why you've chosen the behavior, you can find some compassion for yourself and work towards a more effective strategy.

One strategy you can try is to replace one negative self-medicating behavior for a more positive one. There is still a need for those biochemicals but by finding another alternative, you're getting the benefit of feeling good without the "hangover." By searching for another alternative, you're also in a better position to discover something much more enriching and rewarding while increasing your confidence in your ability to change something you're not quite happy with. Are you ready to find a better solution? Here's your goal.

WEEKLY GOAL

■ What self-medicating behaviors are you currently using? Take a long look at why you do what you do. How often are you shopping? Why are you buying so much? Are you drinking more than you'd like? What's really going on? Discover how you're choosing to self-medicate and discover what it is that you really need. If you're unhappy with your husband, your job, your kids, another pair of shoes won't make everything better. While the best pharmacy is within your own body, this week commit to using the "drugs within" only for your greater good.

Chapter 6
Your Personality

H ave you ever wondered how you're being perceived by those closest to you? We all know that you can't please everyone, but in your search for greater understanding, it may be interesting to discover how your partner, children, extended family, and closest friends describe you. While it may be enlightening, rewarding, or terrifying, it's often a great way to see in yourself what's working and what needs to change.

Every so often, my family plays a game. The game is called "sit in the seat." We each have our own seat at the dinner table. During the game however, we sit in another person's seat and "become that person." We must speak, act, and behave exactly the way the person who usually sits in the seat would behave. While it's mostly fun, it's been horrifying at times to hear back some of the things I've said or ways I've behaved as represented by members of my family. It's also been one of the most significant measures of how I'm being perceived by the people closest to me.

If your loved ones were to describe you, what would they say? This is a great starting point to become the person you want to be. Would they say you always criticize yourself, you have a low self-esteem, and you're always unhappy? Or would they say you're strong, fun, playful, optimistic, easy going and happy? Whatever the characteristics you're hoping to get across don't happen by accident. They occur because those are the messages you're putting out.

Are you making a catastrophe about of everything, where you imagine the worst possible scenario before receiving the results? Are you personalizing where you accept blame and responsibility when it's not your fault? Are you exaggerating where you're making more out of something than need be? Are you labeling someone (or yourself) keeping them from branching outside the label you've set for them? Are you taking things too seriously? Along with other personality traits, these characteristics are just a few that may be revealed with this type of exercise. Good, bad, or otherwise, if the way your loved ones perceive you is less than flattering, you may consider working towards a change.

How about shaking things up a bit and trying to be a little sillier, less task oriented, or more loving? Have you ever seen that look your family gives you when you do something so totally careless, out of character and unexpected? While it throws them off a little, it makes you realize how good it feels, how necessary it is and how happy it makes everyone. With our roles as moms, we infuse ourselves with rules, responsibility, tasks, and chores. Sometimes we become so consumed with our roles, we forget it can be fun too. When I catch myself behaving this way, I usually surprise the family with a puppy. I know it sounds crazy but there's nothing like that look of shock and joy I get from the kids when I bring another one home. Now, I understand this isn't for everyone and I often question it myself so I'll share a few other tips that may work for you.

Every so often, I'll make up a celebration or invent a holiday that we normally don't celebrate. One made up celebration became such a hit that the kids wait for it all year. A few years ago, I realized I was so busy with responsibilities and commitments that I wasn't enjoying as much time with the kids as I could. I also realized I had little time with each one individually. I decided to celebrate half birthdays. These celebrations weren't about parties or gifts, but time alone with me and the half birthday child to do whatever they wanted as long as it was safe and I could be back in time for the other kids. They were allowed to miss school (sorry teachers) and had weeks ahead of time to plan out their special day. They loved that they were excused from following the rules and I got great insight into what they loved to do. Whatever they wanted to do, they got a thrill out of knowing that "responsibility mom" wasn't going to stop them.

Think about opportunities to act silly and look for ways to take on the characteristics you want to have. For example, I remember dragging my daughter from one errand to the next on a cold, rainy day. I was so insistent that she stay dry that I carefully avoided each puddle we came across. At one point I thought "who cares, it's only water." Once making that decision, we ran into each puddle, getting soaked but enjoying our errands along the way.

I have one son who loves Cool Whip. He stared at it longingly in its giant container, looking at me with that resigned look of "oh well." I caught the look and told him to "go for it." He checked with me again. I shook my head yes, and he stuck his entire face into the vat of whipped cream, covering his hair, arms, and legs with the remains. He had so much fun he couldn't wait to tell his friends and made sure Cool Whip was on my next shopping list.

The point is, while these activities are harmless, they're fun and enable you to enjoy your role more fully. Besides enjoying your role, it makes "sit in the seat" a less terrifying game to play. Here's your goal.

WEEKLY GOAL

- How are you being perceived by the people you love the most? Is it flattering and are you being seen the way you want to? If not, you're the only one who can change yourself to be more easy going, lighthearted, comfortable, or secure. Whatever the characteristic you wish to portray, find ways to make it happen. This week, commit to being more spontaneous, impulsive, easy, and fun. Give "responsibility mom" a well earned break as "fun mom" takes over every once in a while. Don't worry you're not slacking off, just searching for a fun, healthy balance.

Chapter 7
Dress To Impress—Yourself

How do you feel when you throw something on, put your hair in a pony tail, wear no makeup, and head out the door? How about when you haven't had a manicure in weeks, your gray hairs are showing, and you're in desperate need of a haircut. Chances are you don't feel as sexy, beautiful, and empowered as you could.

When you take the time to put yourself together, you get an immediate lift in your mood and self-esteem. Think about when you're sick and you stay in bed. The unmade bed may not bother you when you're feeling ill but once you feel better, one of the first things you may want to do is make the bed. The reason is because it makes you feel better. That's what dressing better can offer you as well.

Now, I've already mentioned that I'm no personal stylist or trendsetter when it comes to fashion. What I have learned however is the difference in how a mom can feel when ditching the sweat pants for some well fitting, stylish clothes. I know you want to be comfortable but how about a little less comfort for a more pleasing self-image? I'm not saying you need to prance around in a ball gown and heels, but when you wear something you find flattering, it gives you an instant mood lift. It makes you feel stronger, sexier, more confident, and empowered. Sure there are opportunities for lounging around in sweats but if this is how you're dressing all the time, I'm talking to you.

It doesn't matter if you're overweight. First of all sweats don't hide the weight but accentuate the problem in a number of ways. One way is by preventing you from the positive feeling you get from dressing in more fitted clothing. This feels good and makes you aware of how much better you're able to feel with just a few minor changes. Why deny yourself of that? The other reason is that dressing without care conveys a message that you don't take pride in your appearance.

When something is regarded with value, you handle it with care and take pride in its appearance. For example, picture the stereotypical man who regards his sports car as his "baby." He'll make sure it's clean, wipe it down lovingly, and go through great lengths to make it looks its best because it brings him pride and joy. If he were to neglect the car, you'd view it as not being important, not being as special to him, and not worthy of his time and care. Apply those same ideas to you. When you neglect your appearance, the word is out that you don't value or take pride in yourself. Is that the message you're trying to convey?

It doesn't take a truckload of money to find flattering clothes. What it takes is the desire to change. Even a few new pieces can add a lift to your mood and style while not breaking the bank but first things first. Time for a goal, Cinderella.

WEEKLY GOAL

■ How are you dressing? Are you neglecting your wardrobe due to comfort or your weight? Go into your closet and make some changes. First get rid of anything with holes or stains. Next, give away anything you haven't worn in a year. This will make room for some new things. Try to do this objectively without attaching too much feeling to what you're giving away. After that, keep only a few pieces for "comfort" and donate the rest. Now that you're able to see what you have, it's time to fill in with updated, fitted, more stylish clothing. You may have to leave your comfort zone a little but you can still wear conservative, muted colors if you choose. Whatever your style, the goal is to commit to dressing to impress yourself.

One of the most important concepts to remember in the Emotional Fitness Program Section is that you are in control of your thoughts, behaviors, and reactions. The way you think, feel and act is solely your responsibility and one of the most empowering things you can do for yourself is to accept that responsibility fully. By accepting responsibility for yourself you are in the driver's seat as opposed to being a passenger on your journey through life. You control your thoughts, which control your behaviors, which control your reactions to what you see around you. By accepting responsibility you are in a proactive position rather than a reactive position, directing your life as opposed to simply reacting to it. Just imagine what you're doing for your emotional outlook when you understand that you are in control of every emotion you feel!

Please understand that I'm not saying that changing your outlook means you'll never experience negative emotion. Not only is it normal to feel sad, lonely, upset, or aggravated from time to time but it's healthy. The problem arises once you've experienced the emotion. What do you do with it? How do you react and how do you feel afterwards? These are the feelings that you control and with a plan, effort and energy, you can retrain yourself to react in any way you choose. There's no "I couldn't help it," "He made me feel this way," or "It's all her fault." No one steps on you without your permission and no one has the power to control your thoughts but you. Take hold of that power, that responsibility and that insight to steer yourself whichever way you choose!

Relationship
Fitness Program

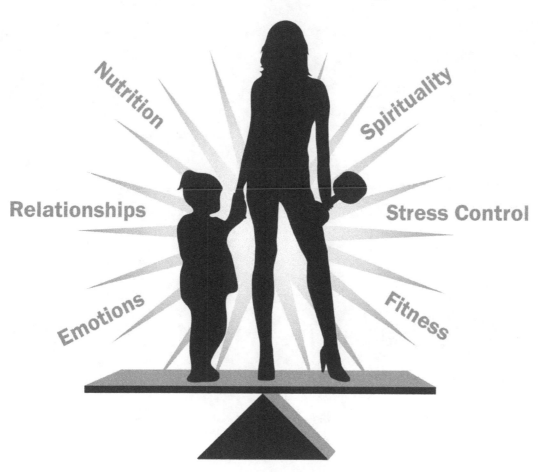

Introduction

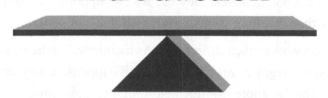

Tell me who you spend your time with and I'll tell you how you feel. Sounds impossible? It's really not. You see, we often take on the feelings, behaviors, and attitudes of those we spend time with. For example, let's say you have a friend or coworker who's always complaining. She's speaks negatively about her body, her job, her relationships, and her life. She looks forward to spending time with you because it gives her an opportunity to vent and find relief. Once she's through, she feels lighter, freer, and ready to go on with her day. She enjoys speaking to you because you're a great listener, enabling her to be heard and valued. That works for her, but how do you feel? Chances are you feel drained, deflated, and uninspired. Although your intention was to be a good friend, once you became involved emotionally in your friends negativity, you were brought right down with her.

Now on the other hand, let's say you have plans to see a friend who is lighthearted, enthusiastic, and embraces life with eagerness and zest. Just thinking about this friend brings a smile to your face because you know you'll be having fun and enjoying each other's company. After your time together, you're excited about the rest of your day. You want to capture every moment and see all the beauty that's around you. Your friend may not have intentionally tried to alter your thinking but her positive approach and attitude was infectious.

Which person is better for your health? Studies show that positive thinkers have a 55 percent lower risk of death from all causes and 33 percent lower risk of death from heart failure. That's not to say that the more positive person doesn't experience anything unpleasant. In fact, the positive, optimistic person may have experienced more unfortunate situations than the negative, pessimistic person. The result of these experiences however leaves the positive thinker with a greater appreciation, perspective, and sense of gratitude. They are grateful for what they see and have because they may have something less pleasant to compare it with.

When they encounter a stressful situation, they look for ways to improve it versus letting it consume them. When a problem arises, they use it as an opportunity to find the most appropriate solution, rather than dwelling or magnifying all that's gone wrong.

The negative person works much differently. As mentioned in the Emotional Fitness Program Section, they expect negative results and when it happens, it only confirms what they'd originally predicted. They're more comfortable judging, gossiping, or criticizing because putting others down offers them some relief from their pain. The negative person maintains the role of "victim" in a script she's written for herself. She feels other's are responsible for her "lot in life" and often uses it as an excuse to stay exactly where she is.

Within each of us is a broad range of emotions. An optimist doesn't only experience joy and the pessimist doesn't only experience negativity. It's just that the optimist chooses to expect happiness, success, and pleasure and as a result, that's what they find. The pessimist chooses to replay negative thoughts which lead to negative results. It's a choice. We choose how we want to think, feel, and act. Although we may be conditioned to think or react a certain way, if we don't like the results it is our choice to change. That's why if we're working towards changing the way we think, feel, and react, it's important to be careful about the people you're spending your time with. Look for like minded people who support, encourage, and inspire you. Limit your time with people who drain, upset, and frustrate you.

This is your life. You are the driver of your car on the road to fulfillment, greater purpose, and happiness. While there may be many detours, you have the power to steer yourself in whichever direction you choose to go. If you want to feel good, steer yourself towards an optimistic perspective and let your relationships support your cause. If you choose pessimism, misery loves company, and you'll find many people welcoming you into their negative club. Life is a journey and we don't travel alone. Who are you bringing on your ride?

Throughout this section, we'll be focusing on many different aspects of relationships. It's so important because our relationships define us. They offer a glimpse into what we're about, what we stand for, what we tolerate, and what we expect. We'll cover how our relationships are affecting our body, mind, and spirit. We'll talk about how we teach others how to treat us by the way we treat ourselves (uh oh!). We'll discuss the importance of integrity, intentions, setting boundaries, mindful speech, and mindful listening in order to bring our relationships to a higher level. We'll cover how to recognize and deal with those who steal your energy, zap you of your strength, burst your bubble, criticize, judge, blame, discourage, and deflate you. Finally, we'll talk about how to begin, enhance, and enjoy our relationships by improving the way we speak, listen, and understand those around us. We have a lot to cover. Are you ready?

Chapter 1
Your Relationships and Your Health

I t's hard to believe that your relationships actually determine your health but study after study shows it to be true. One study was done by Duke University. Results of the study showed that the positive feelings such as feelings of belonging and togetherness actually strengthened the immune system in study participants.

Another study showed how colds and viruses were more likely in those with few relationships and social interactions. This happened because the immune system was found to be suppressed in those with few relationships and the infection had a chance to enter and upset the body.

In yet another study, it was found that moms of young children who felt they had no emotional support were three times at risk for mental health problems as opposed to moms who received emotional support. These moms had no one who could offer support, share ideas, or simply vent their frustration to, leaving mom to feel isolated and alone.

Finally, a study with breast cancer patients compared the length of time the breast cancer went into remission by studying two groups of patients, one with support and one without support. The study found that the group of breast cancer patients receiving support had a remission eighteen months longer than the group without support! What does this mean?

It means that the support we receive from the relationships we have offers us protection against illness and disease. Support strengthens our immune system, provides healthy outlets for our stress and reduces the level of unhealthy stress chemicals floating around within our bodies. Our bodies have a chance to re-balance, heal, and work normally without the added wear and tear that isolation, rejection, or being in few or dysfunctional relationships can cause.

What type of relationships do you have? Before we can change how we feel or behave in the relationships we have, we need to learn more about who we're spending our time, energy, and effort on. You guessed it, time for a goal.

WEEKLY GOAL

- This week, write down who you spend your time with and in what capacity (kids, spouse, work, friend, volunteer, etc.). Next to each name, make a plus sign (+) or minus sign (–) when determining how they make you feel (most of the time). If being with these people enhances your well being, give them a plus sign. If being with these people fills you with negativity, self-doubt, hurt, anger, or frustration, give them a minus sign. Next, see how many plus signs you have, how many minus signs you have. We need to work on how we handle the relationships with the minus signs, while increasing the time we spend with the relationships with the plus signs. This week, commit to discovering how your relationships make you feel.

Chapter 2
What Types of Relationships Do You Have?

Now that you know where the pluses and the minuses are coming from, it's time to evaluate each one. I always like to get the bad news out of the way so lets start with the minuses first.

One of the reasons we tolerate being mistreated is due to a low self-esteem. We feel less deserving or worthy somehow and use that to determine the quality of relationships we can hope for and expect. Think about it. How would your relationships be different if you felt better about yourself? Would you expect more respect, support, sincerity, intimacy, honesty, compassion?

As I've said, we teach others how to treat us. If we speak negatively about ourselves, criticize, judge, or label ourselves, it's only natural that others will due the same. We're showing them a step-by-step plan of how to disrespect us following our own example. Maybe speaking about yourself this way is an old habit that you've had for years. Well, bad habits are meant to be replaced by good ones and this one's worth changing.

I'm not implying that it's completely your responsibility that there are mean or disrespectful people in your life. In fact, very often those are the ones who provide you with the greatest life lessons because they teach you how *not* to be while setting a clear example of something better you may want for yourself. They are often a catalyst to changing something in your life so while your experiences may be upsetting, if you're able to use the lessons learned in your favor, it often leads you on a path to your better self. For example, let's say you grew up in a dysfunctional home. Your parents were abusive and you were raised in an unloving environment. While traumatic, you have two choices. You can either continue into your adult years with what you've learned or use the experiences to enable you to become a loving, attentive parent. Of course it's hard to "undo" the damage but as I've said already, nothing really good comes easy. Plus, the reward of discontinuing this cycle is one of the best gifts you can give to your children—and yourself (if this is too difficult of a process for you alone, get the support you need).

Without having those negative relationships, you'd never appreciate how much nicer, sweeter, more appreciative, or loving a healthy relationship can be. Negative relationships offer that comparison for you to determine what you want and need. So although some relationships can exhaust you, look for the bigger picture as to what they provide and you'll slowly move on from that greater awareness. There are no mistakes. Every person in our life is there for a reason. Whether it's to learn greater patience, self-control, or compassion it's our job to take the lesson being taught and learn from it. Time for a goal.

WEEKLY GOAL

- This week, commit to determining what life lesson each of your stressful relationships provide. There's a lesson under all that frustration. Next, evaluate if some of your negative relationships (an obnoxious co-worker, neighbor, etc.) is worthy of continuing. It's often helpful to write it down. Fold a piece of paper in half writing the positives you get from the relationship on one side and the negatives you get from the relationship on the other. If you find that the relationship is providing more pain than pleasure, determine if it's worth continuing. If not, decide on the most respectful, tactful and kind way to break the news.

Chapter 3
What Negative Relationships Do To Your Body

If you've already been through the Stress Control Fitness Program or the Emotional Control Fitness Program, you've had a glimpse in to what negative feelings can do to your physical health. Here's a quick summary in case you haven't gone through those programs yet.

Every thought (good or bad) has a biochemical response attached to it. That means that microscopic chemicals are released according to the thought you just had. When you have a happy thought, "feel good" chemicals are released that have been found to nourish, support, and heal the body. When you have a negative thought, "stress hormones" are released. They were designed as an effective means to get you out of harms way. For example, if a car were quickly approaching, the release of these chemicals enables your body to immediately jump onto the curb to safety. It's a protective mechanism, designed for use over the short term.

These same chemicals are released when you have a negative thought. The problem is, they're released but never turned off. So consider "jumping the curb to safety." Your heart's pounding, you start to sweat, pupils dilate, etc. After a few minutes, your body has a chance to calm down and return to normal. When we have these negative thoughts (from our dysfunctional or destructive relationships) these chemicals are released with no end in sight. Over time, the depletion of these chemicals causes huge bodily wear and tear. You know how you feel so drained and *worn out* when dealing with negative people? That's *exactly* what we're allowing them to do to us.

Okay. So I've given you the bad news and what do you do now? You may think "I've had a horrible relationship with my (fill in the blank) for years. I can't just end it. I just have to suffer through." Well, it's certainly your right to make that decision. If that is your decision, here's an idea…

First and foremost, the only person you can change is yourself. Throughout my almost twenty years working exclusively with moms, I've found many moms frustrated with their inability to change their husbands, kids, parents, etc. Part of that frustration ends when you understand that just as you can only change yourself, the other person can only change themselves too (and that's only if they think *they* need to!). So, starting from this understanding you can now make some headway.

While you can't change a person, you can change the way you interpret, respond, and react to them. I'll give you a classic example. One of my children had temper tantrums every morning before school from age two to age four. For about twenty minutes, he'd be kicking, screaming, pounding on the walls, floor, pillows, stuffed animals, basically anything he could get his hands on. It was incredibly frustrating. For one, I was overscheduled with my morning tasks so "there wasn't time" for his outbursts. Secondly, he saw that, tantrum or not, we still went to his kiddie class, preschool, whatever, so why didn't he just give this up already?

This is the interesting part. What happened more often that not was that the angrier he became, the more frustrated I became. He'd start his tantrum, I'd get frustrated. Although I tried talking, holding, explaining as a way to get him to stop, this was a part of the morning routine for two long years. What also made it so intolerable was the fact that I had other kids needing me and dogs barking for attention. What's the point to this story?

One day, I decided not to react. I promised myself that I wouldn't take it personally, wouldn't feel defeated, frustrated, or any other "bad mom" feeling and would just take his tantrum in stride. His tantrums were so predictable and exasperating that I got myself ready minutes before "show time." As expected, he started screaming and I didn't react. In fact, I just started laughing at the craziness of it all. It finally got to me that for two years, this was how we spent our mornings! You can't even imagine the look on my other kids faces when they thought "mom's really lost it now."

After a few minutes, the craziest thing happened. My red faced, screaming son slowly realized he'd lost his audience. He wasn't getting the expected reaction, the crazed mom (me) wasn't reacting and his tantrums just weren't working anymore. Not only was mom not going crazy but she was laughing! Well, after a few minutes, guess who started laughing too?! Soon enough, we were having a good time! I finally realized (to my horror) that good or bad, he was mimicking me! So when he was having his tantrum, I was providing the necessary fuel for the fire! The only part that made it not so funny was when I realized the physical damage I must have caused myself over the last two years!

While this story has a happy ending, I'm sure there are people in your life who are equally exasperating with no end in sight (we all have them). For these people, it's simply a matter of deciding that you won't let them deeply affect you. Whether you envision a coat of armor around you that they can't penetrate with their negativity, imagining you're partially hard of hearing when they're speaking with disrespect, or reminding yourself that when they upset you, it's causing you bodily distress. Choose whichever strategy you're most comfortable with and start protecting your body, mind, and spirit.

There's also a trick one of my clients used. She had a terrible problem with one of her relatives. This relative treated her horribly, often criticizing, belittling, humiliating, and judging whenever he felt it appropriate. Her rational side understood that it was his problem, a deep insecurity and a feeling that he wasn't liked, wanted, or valued. Unfortunately, the other part of her couldn't justify taking the abuse but felt she had no choice. Whenever this relative spoke, she imagined (get ready) that she was talking to a monkey! She actually pictured him standing there like a baboon swinging from a tree. Now, if a monkey were to make crazy noises at you would you get offended, angry, upset? That's exactly why this technique worked so well for her. You guessed it, time for a goal.

WEEKLY GOAL

- Let's say you know which relationships are causing you frustration, you understand that it's up to you to change how you react to it, and you're willing to come up with a strategy. Complaining about it is pointless unless it brings you to a decision about how to deal or react with this person. Wallowing in it only causes you physical harm (which may make you feel worse once you realize the offending person is bothering you and causing you physical wear and tear). So it's time for a plan. What's your strategy for the next interaction with this person? What will you do to not take the words personally, feel the hurt or pain the person is trying to cause? Will you limit your time with this person or find another way to make it work for you? This week, commit to finding an effective means to deal with this person in order to limit the "damage" it causes you.

Speaking of limiting your time with this person, this is often an effective strategy that you may want to try. Let's say you have a "frienemy" that's a friend who's not really looking out for your best interest. Often, she can't help herself; she wants to be a good friend but hasn't learned or mastered the necessary skills. You don't always have to be available and you don't always have to provide a reason why. This person may take the hint, or if you want, you may need to sit them down and explain that your friendship has changed.

Chapter 4
Creating and Setting Boundaries

Another reason relationships get into the trouble zone is because we fail to set boundaries as to what we're willing to tolerate. People often do (or not do) what they can get away with. You've probably noticed this with your kids. Maybe you've asked them to clean their room. It's not done immediately and they're kind of waiting to see if they can get away with watching TV instead. If you let it go, you've just shown them that it's okay to disrespect your wishes, no big deal. They tested your boundaries and got away with it pretty easily. Now let's say you ask them again. They'll probably wait to see how seriously you mean it. If they can get away with not responding to your request, they probably will. See what's going on here?

I'm not saying that your kids aren't wonderful. I'm sure they are. What I'm saying is that your boundaries are being tested to see how strong and firm they are. You determine this and no one else. If you don't like the set up that's been created, it's up to you to change. Think about how your boundaries have been crossed and how you've responded. Do you feel violated, disrespected, or not taken seriously when your needs are expressed? Now, I'm not a psychologist nor do I pretend to be. I can only share with you what I've seen over the years along with my own knowledge and experience. One conclusion that's safe to say is that if something's working for you, great. If it's not working (and you know it's not by the way you feel) it's worth looking into another solution.

The more we respect ourselves, the more respect we give others and the more we expect to be treated respectfully. The more we love ourselves, the more love we give and the more love we typically get in return. See what's going on here? It starts and ends with us. How we feel about ourselves, how we view ourselves and how we treat ourselves is the "lesson plan" for others to follow. Now, for many of us, we may not even be aware of how we're being viewed, how we speak and how we sound. We may cringe if we actually knew how our messages were being interpreted by others. One way to avoid misunderstandings, miscommunications, and fiery confrontations is by mindfully listening and mindfully speaking. What do I mean?

Let's start with mindfully listening. This begins with the understanding that both you and whoever you're talking to both want to be happy. You both want to be treated with respect, understood, valued, and heard. There is no assuming you know anything because you can't know what's going on inside someone else's mind. You also have to listen carefully to the tone, watch the body language, and ask enough questions so you don't form the answers from your perspective. This is where we often go wrong. We know how we feel in certain situations and assume the other person is feeling the same thing. We jump to conclusions and often miss the boat entirely. We also fail to listen long enough for the person to fully explain their position.

Another sign that we're not mindfully listening is when we become defensive. This is when the hearing stops and we're trying to cover up and protect ourselves. Without mindful listening, the person feels cheated, cut off, devalued and unhappy. The best way to mindfully listen is to wait until you're both calm, stop what you're doing, look the person in the eyes, listen without judgment and the hardest part of all…just listen. You'd be amazed at what you can learn and what you've finally allowed yourself to hear.

Mindfully speaking is different. This involves a few key things that many people find difficult to do. The first is taking responsibility. That means saying "I" instead of "you." For example, instead of saying "You made me so angry" you say "I feel angry." You're not blaming, you're explaining how you feel. Speaking mindfully also means that we fully understand our motivation and intentions. Is there another way something may be interpreted? Is that sarcasm really your way of hurting one another? What did you *really* mean behind what you said? Are your intentions "above board" when you're speaking, or is there a hidden agenda? Only you know these answers and you control every word that leaves your mouth, good or bad. It's often helpful when you look at it like this; your words are a verbal interpretation of how you feel about yourself. Kind, loving, honest words flow from someone secure, comfortable, and at peace with themselves. Harsh, critical, judgmental words come from someone often lacking those feelings. How are your boundaries? Are you mindfully listening? Mindfully speaking? Here's your goal.

WEEKLY GOAL

■ This week, determine if your boundaries are set where you want them to be. Are you happy with the results they bring? If not, they need to be changed. Next, try to get a better sense of how you're speaking and listening. If you were on the receiving end of your words, how would you feel? Would someone feel heard after talking with you? If not, why? Could you be misinterpreting someone's message by the way you're (not) hearing them? How can your speaking and listening be changed to avoid miscommunication? You may also find that you speak differently according to who you're speaking with. Take note of your intentions. Again, you can't change how someone else speaks or listens. What you can change is your half of the exchange and as they say, "that's half the battle."

Chapter 5
The Limiting Label

L et's talk about labels. Maybe you were always "the smart one," "the pretty one," "the shy one," "the athlete," "the geek," "the clown," and the list goes on and on. The labels may have been flattering or may have been demeaning. In either case, chances are you lived up to the label you were given. It's part of the legacy we leave childhood with. Think about it. Let's say you were "the smart one." You probably got showered with praise and attention when you did anything intelligent. This felt good so you kept at it in order to receive that praise. But what happened when you wanted to be silly or creative in a way that was new to you? Chances are you didn't take the risk. Why? The praise you were receiving from being "the smart one" felt good and venturing into the unknown wasn't worth the risk of being criticized, questioned, or losing that status.

Even though a label may be flattering, it's limiting because it often prevents you from stepping out of that comfort zone of how you're being viewed and received. We fail to strive beyond our labels. Without the label, all areas are fair game as there are no expectations of how you *should* behave. Now, people love to categorize people, places, and things. It may be a way for us to organize and compartmentalize things mentally when we know what category everything belongs in. So maybe you grew up in a home with a few siblings. Each of you got your own label and it served as a way to easily describe you. While it may have described you, think of how it may have held you back.

Now, consider a negative label we may have been given, or a label we may have interpreted to be negative. When it was said enough times, we probably just accepted it to be true. This is exactly how our belief systems are formed. It's nothing more than someone we trust (or a group, organization, society, etc.) saying the same thing with conviction over and over again. We eventually buy into it and it becomes part of our belief system. Think about it. When you look at your belief system, what are your beliefs based on? Repetition of an idea from someone you trust.

Now here's the bad news. Let's say the person we trusted was on the receiving end of some limiting beliefs themselves. As a result, while they may not have meant to, they may have unintentionally passed that damage on to you. They most probably meant no harm but they instilled a belief on you with a label (good or bad). Because of your trust and belief in that person of authority, it became your belief as well. For example, let's say you had a parent who always called you "lazy." Maybe they were trying to motivate you to be another way or maybe they felt it was an accurate description of how you behaved. In either case, you grew up thinking "if they said it all those times, it must be true." So when opportunities came up, you heard that ongoing tape in your head "you're lazy" and figured that whatever was involved may take too much effort for you because you're just too lazy.

Here's the upside. You can get rid of all of these limiting beliefs once you identify them, evaluate them, and decide to discard them. Just as I keep saying, it's our job to change whatever we don't like. As I've also said, it may not be easy, but it's so worth it. Want to start with a new label without any limits? Okay, you're the wonderful one making all those great lifestyle changes. Here's your goal.

WEEKLY GOAL

- Think about all of the labels you have along with labels you may have placed on others. Are they limiting in any way? Chances are they've prevented you and others from venturing outside the existing label. This week, determine the labels you've been given and the labels you've given to others. See where they've prevented you from thinking, acting, or behaving in a way that may have been satisfying, enriching, or fulfilling. Determine how they've held you back. Understand that your belief in that label is nothing more than repetition of someone else's idea that we bought into. Don't hold the person responsible for the label;

they didn't know any better. The best way to stop punishing yourself for going through years with a negative label is rewarding yourself by discontinuing this learned behavior onto someone else. Now, for any label you don't like, decide that it's time to discard them. Realize that you can buy into them if you want to or discard them if you don't, it's your choice.

Chapter 6
Judgment, Criticism and Jealousy

D o you have people in your life who judge you? These are the people who determine if what you do or say is right or wrong. First of all, who gave them this
power? Secondly, how does it make you feel?

When we became moms, we sure weren't handed a step-by-step guide on how to raise
our kids (although it may have been helpful!). Through trial and error, we navigated our
way by learning what works best for us and our family. Our decisions may have been based
on what we learned from others, what we grew up with (or not) ourselves, what felt right,
and what supports our values and beliefs. We may have been afraid, insecure, or cautious
regarding the decisions we made but eventually, we figured out some ways to make it work.
Now, when we're feeling insecure about a decision we need to make or just made, and we're
judged by someone we've given this power to, what happens?

First of all judgment squelches our creativity and individuality. It's a way of making
us uncomfortable with the choices we're making because we assume the person judging us
knows better than we do. The more insecure we are with our decision, the more judgment
from others affects us. That's why it's easy to see how a new mom is so easily influenced
by the judgment from others. She's venturing into an unknown territory, insecure with her
ability in this new role, and is easily influenced by someone who's already been in her posi-

tion. Well, I'm going to ask you something. Just because someone else was a new mom at one point, does that mean that her decisions are automatically better than yours may be? Her decisions were based on her prior experiences, conditioning, and influence by others. That doesn't automatically make the same decision right for you. Also, many people who judge are judging you because they've found flaws in their own choices. They're uncomfortable with the results their decisions have brought, and they pass that insecurity on to you.

Another characteristic that can get in the way of relationships is criticism. Why does someone criticize? Is it helpful? Often, the person criticizing takes the position of "I'm only trying to help." What's important here is to clearly understand the person's intentions behind the comments. If they're just terrible with words, it may be worth discussing some better word choices that wouldn't seem as offensive. If the intention is to hurt, embarrass, or belittle you, you may want to consider where this anger is coming from. Was there a miscommunication and an unresolved conflict that could easily be cleared up? Is there underlying resentment from someone with an unmet need you've provided in the past? Possible reasons for criticism can be endless. What's important is to get to the bottom of it so you can both speak clearly and respectfully to one another.

Let's talk about jealousy. Jealousy is an important characteristic to be aware of because it's so telling. If we're jealous, it shows us what it is that we want and don't have. We need to evaluate these feelings to see if they're justified and if we're willing to do what it takes to get what it is that we obviously want. Is it possible, logical, or reasonable? Is it something we want badly enough, or would we rather just complain about not having it?

For example, I've worked with hundreds of moms who complain about their bodies. They hate how they look, they're uncomfortable with the way they feel, and they're jealous of anyone who has a stronger, leaner, and more fit body than they have. That's when I usually ask "So, what do you want to do about it?" I then usually hear "she probably never eats any chocolate," or "she probably spends all day in the gym." I don't say a word. Finally, the truth comes out "I don't want to work that hard!" Well, at least they were honest. The jealousy served a purpose because it showed them what they want…but may not be willing to work for!

Once you understand this, it's easier to not get upset or offended when others are jealous of you. It truly is a form of flattery (although it rarely feels like it) because you clearly have something that someone else wants. Using our same scenario from above, a more confident and secure person would probably just go right up to the thin, fit person and say "you look great, what do you do to stay so fit?" They would also quickly realize that they have no right to be jealous if they're not willing to put in the same effort and commitment. Sounds about right? Are you dealing with judgment, criticism and jealousy? Time for your goal.

WEEKLY GOAL

- We're focusing on judgment, criticism, and jealousy here and we're going to handle it from two perspectives. First, decide if you are passing judgment, criticism, or having feelings of jealousy in some of the relationships you have. Why do you feel this way? What is it doing to your relationships and how can you change? What is the underlying feeling you have that is showing itself in these destructive ways? Get to the bottom of it and make the decision that you're ready to change. It truly will change the quality of any relationship you have. Next, determine who is judging, criticizing, and acting jealous towards you. How is it showing itself? Are you willing to respectfully confront this person and find out what's going on? Are these relationships worth it to you? Is it time to let go? Only you know these answers. This week, commit to discovering the truth about judgment, criticism, and jealousy from your end and from those in your life. Determine the quality of the relationship with these characteristics in play and decide if things would be better another way. You know what's best for you. Trust yourself.

Chapter 7
Respect

Have you ever noticed how with some people, you simply want to be your best? It has nothing to do with what the person does or says specifically, but there's just something about this person that makes you strive to be better, especially when you're around them. Think about if there are any people like this in your life. Maybe it's a mentor, religious leader, spiritual leader, coworker, friend, mail carrier, or supermarket cashier. It doesn't matter what they do. What matters is how they make you feel.

Whether they're caring, generous, lighthearted, intuitive, or just friendly, there's some quality they have that brings out your best. If you have these people in your life, consider yourself blessed. Learn all you can from their warm, infectious spirit. If you don't have people like this in your life, try and find them.

The next thing to think about is why you find these people so pleasing? Chances are you'll find that these special individuals like and respect you for exactly who you are. They make no judgments about what you do or say, figuring only you know what's best for you. Around them, you feel valued, heard, understood, and appreciated. You feel connected, approved, and most of all, respected for who you are. Do not take this lesson lightly moms. I'm a full believer in copying something if it feels right (as long as you give the teacher credit—which they'll very humbly accept). These people come into your life providing rich examples of characteristics to embrace. If you like something, you can take it on and with practice, make it your own. It's like buying a new pair of shoes. At first they might be uncomfortable, but over time, they'll feel like they were made to fit.

So often we put our behavior on autopilot, never striving to change the way we think or react. We often put more effort into choosing an outfit than evaluating personality traits that need tweaking. We may also spend precious time explaining, defending, and proving ourselves when involved in certain relationships. This tiresome activity only leaves us to question our own worth. We can spend decades this way without even questioning why we put ourselves through this.

If you like a trait or not, you'll know by how you feel. Let your feelings be your guide as to what is best for your health and wellness. Some people enjoy competition, control, perfection, and aggression. They seek out these characteristics and make them their own. For others, a kind, gentle, respectful approach is the best way to go. What's important is that you surround yourself with people who have qualities you like and want for yourself. Being around these positive qualities is the first step to making them your own. Are there qualities you see that you like enough to take on? When you picture yourself at your best, what qualities do you possess? Time for a goal.

WEEKLY GOAL

- When it comes to this goal, imitation is flattery. Think about a person you know who has qualities that make you feel good. Why do you feel good when you're with this person? Are they sweet, sensitive, lighthearted, fun, or intuitive? What is it about this person that makes you feel respected, secure, and calm? This week, commit to discovering which qualities and characteristics you want to take on and make your own. It's okay to copy as long as you give the teacher credit. Mentors, teachers, and guides are all around us. It's in our best interest to open up our eyes and hearts and take in all the good stuff.

Chapter 8
Dating Your Spouse

I f you're like many moms, the sexiest thing your husband may tell you is: "go to bed honey, I've got the kids." While children may bring you joy, satisfaction and fulfill-ment, they can easily suck the spark from your marriage, if you let them. Now, I'm going to say something that may shock you, may come as a surprise, or may just be some-thing you hadn't thought of. Are you ready?

One day, whether it's now or in the next twenty years, your children will leave the nest you raised them in. They will be ready, willing, and able to fly on their own because of all of the love, nurturing and support you've supplied. They will have plans, dreams, and minds of their own (which hopefully you can find a way to agree with for your own sanity). If you do nothing to nurture your relationship with your spouse now, when your kids leave, you will be slammed with a harsh reality of "uh oh, what now." You may then also look at your spouse and think "who is this guy?" You may even take it a step further and think "I haven't spoken to him in years. Do I even like this person?"

My in-laws, who will be renewing their vows as part of a huge fiftieth wedding anni-versary party the kids and grandkids are throwing for them this year told me something I'll never forget many years ago. I'd always admired the way they spoke and acted towards one another. Always holding hands, kissing each other hello and goodbye, I wanted to know their secret for lasting success as I became engaged to their son. I remember asking my mother-in-law the question, "What can I do so that I want to hold my husband's hand years from now?" My mother-in-law looked at me and said "Just by *wanting* to you're halfway there." She also said, "Your kids will come and go, so in order to like who you're looking at when they leave make every effort to *always* stay close."

This leads to my next point about the importance of dating your spouse. What do I mean? Remember how you wanted to impress each other when you first started to date? You always wanted to look good, say nice things and you always found interest in what each other had to say. Are you still trying to impress each other? Do you both still try to put yourselves together, smell nice, and say kind words to each other? Do you have a relationship *outside* of your children?

We get so caught up in our daily lives that it's easy to just update each other on the basics and forget the rest. We're often so exhausted from our schedules that an extra hour of sleep seems far more appealing than reconnecting with each other. Finally, many of us feel that once the vows have been made, the effort stops.

It's so easy to go your separate ways once you have children. You become so deeply entrenched in motherhood that you forget you're a woman too. You've given so much all day that by the time you see your husband, there's nothing left to give. You're exhausted, spent, depleted, and want nothing more than a good night's rest. Here's what's going on from his perspective.

He's overwhelmed too. He has stress from his day and looks to unwind and recharge by coming home after work. When he walks in the door however, instead of the June Cleaver scenario he may have secretly been hoping for, he's met by a wife who may not have found time to shower, screaming kids, and a hectic, chaotic scene. He knows how overwhelmed things are, so it's useless to point it out. It's easier for him to be quietly unhappy than ruffle your feathers. What does this lead to?

This often leads to mutually agreeable coexistence. That's my term for when a husband and wife each have their own roles, coexist within the home, and blandly make it work. While this is often how many couples live, it doesn't have to be this way. For one, at one point you were attracted to each other. So, whatever that initial attraction was, this is what you may want to rediscover within each other again.

The next point is, if you're going to go through your days with this person, raising a family, and spending time, effort, and energy, why not make it as pleasurable as you can? The days will come and go. You're not getting them back so why not reach for something better within your marriage? It can be blah or it can be great; it's up to the two of you.

The last point is, your children look at the two of you to see how you get along. This is how they determine what they need to do when they enter into relationships. Your daughter will learn how she should expect to be treated from a man, her role within a relationship, and how she should feel within a marriage. Your son will look at his dad to determine how to treat a woman, his role within a relationship, and how to behave within a marriage. Do you like what they're learning? If not, it's up to the two of you to make some changes.

So, let's say things have gotten out of hand. You've put your relationship on the back burner, and you've noticed that there's plenty of room for improvement. What can you do?

Just as when you want any change to last, start small. Come up with a few ideas together and then come up with a few on your own. Have your spouse come up with a few of his own too. Look for ways to compliment each other, surprise, or impress each other. One of the biggest problems I see with the moms I work with is that they think changes have to be monumental to make a difference. They don't. Something subtle like a simple compliment can work wonders. You both need them and it just feels good. Daily "mini-connections" like a gentle touch or private conversation are a few other ways to stay close. Do kind acts you know the other would appreciate like making his favorite meal or have him bring you your morning cup of coffee. All it takes is the desire to make it better. Of course you're tired, overwhelmed, stressed, etc. So is he, but that doesn't mean you neglect each other and hope for the best. The stronger you are as a team, the better it is for everyone. As I've said so many times already, nothing really good comes easy, but isn't a great marriage worth the effort? Here's your goal.

WEEKLY GOAL

- If your marriage has lost its sizzle, this goal's for you. This week, commit to doing something nice for each other every day. It can be something as simple as a smile when each other enters the room or anything as elaborate as (you fill in the blank...be creative here). The goal is to find a way to "date" again. That means you still want to impress each other, still respect, like, and want to be together. Think back to that initial attraction, what drew you towards each other in the first place and try to bring that back. Get a babysitter (hire one once a week, trade babysitting services with a friend) so you have time to reconnect. Get out of the house and do something fun. Find a hobby, sport, or activity you can do together and make it your "special time." Make it a priority to get back the spark you once had for each other. Keep trying and let each other know what works and what doesn't. Happy dating!

Chapter 9
When it's Time to End Relationships—Forgiveness and Letting Go

Each of us has a boiling point. We each have a threshold that lets us know if we aren't willing to continue with a relationship for one reason or another. Maybe you feel violated, disrespected, unappreciated, taken advantage of, misunderstood, hurt, or abused. For whatever reason, sometimes toxic relationships get to a point where it's more painful to be in them than out of them.

No one can be the judge of this but you. Only you know what you're willing to accept. So often we're sleepwalking through our lives and this causes unhealthy relationships to simply continue. When we're exposed to an alternative or just decide to wake up and "smell the coffee," we often discover that a toxic relationship no longer has a place in our desire for a healthy, fulfilling life. For many, this reality causes panic, denial, and the refusal to accept that changes need to be made. For others, it becomes apparent that the destructive relationship we're in has been holding us back from discovering our best selves. We feel we've come so far, we can't turn back, and the toxic relationship puts our healing, growth, happiness, and emotional well being at great risk.

As I've said earlier, every relationship serves a purpose even if that relationship showed you nothing more than what you *don't* want in the future. Crazy as it seems, these people are often our best teachers because they make what we *do* want so clear.

Staying in any dysfunctional, toxic relationship can leave us questioning our self-worth, self-esteem, and better judgment. It can leave you feeling depressed, anxious, angry, resentful, and unhappy. Walking around with these feelings over time is damaging to our health due to the over secretion of hormones from these negative emotions we constantly feel. Now, I'm not saying that relationships (kids, parents, spouses, friends, etc.) don't go through difficult periods. We change, along with the people and circumstances in our lives, all the time. When this occurs, it requires the relationship to change and grow as well. Adjustments need to be made, new boundaries need to be set, and the relationship grows in a new and different direction. This is all normal and expected.

Unfortunately however, some relationships are unable to withstand the inevitable change that growth, development, and greater awareness brings. For example, the relationship may have worked because someone was manipulative and controlling and you lacked the confidence to stand your ground. Once you gained that ability, the other person felt threatened because your improved self-esteem required that the rules within the relationship needed to change.

Another example of when relationships may not be able to be saved is when you've had a painful past and you've finally found the courage, strength, and ability to break free. At some point you may become aware that the pain, anguish, and poor self-esteem you suffered as a result of being the brunt of someone else's problems wasn't worth the suffering anymore. You may feel the relationship caused you to pay too big a price and you're not willing to let it hold you back or cause any further damage to your emotional, physical, or spiritual health. You may realize the destruction it's caused in your perception of what a normal, healthy relationship could be. Finally, you may find that once you gather the strength to end a painful chapter of your life it gives you an opportunity to heal, grow, and open the door to something wonderfully unexpected.

As I've said, only you know if a relationship needs tweaking, a complete overhaul, or if it finally needs to end. If you do find that your relationship is beyond repair it is often a painful discovery. It can be painful on so many levels and for so many reasons. It will take time to accept, implement, and adjust. But if it was the right choice, you'll find that as difficult as it is, you're better off mentally, physically, emotionally, and spiritually by breaking free. Of course, get the help and support you need to get you through. If you've "had enough of having enough" it may be time for you to begin the process of cutting the ties and begin the healing process. But again, no one knows if it's time but you.

Now, in order for you to truly move on from a dysfunctional and destructive relationship, one of the most important concepts you may want to consider is forgiveness. Forgiveness is an incredibly personal and individual thing. We each have our own definition and criteria of what we're willing to forgive, how we're willing to forgive, and at what point we're willing to forgive.

Some people feel that the only way to move on from something painful is to actually forgive the person who hurt you. You may or may not agree with this. Here's my interpretation. When I say that forgiveness is important, I'm talking about releasing yourself from the power the pain has had over you. We can go decades harboring grudges, resentment, and pain. It can show itself in excess weight, poor health, and low self-esteem. The longer we hold onto our pain, the more power the person who hurt you still has. I always think about this example used by Dr. Wayne Dyer. He explains pain and suffering by comparing it to a snake bite. It's not the snake bite that kills you but the venom that's released. That venom is released by us. Yes the snake did the biting but the constant replay of the bite is within our control.

Letting go of that hurt can be one of the most freeing and liberating things you ever do. I've seen moms able to drop weight they've struggled with for years, put an end to a digestive problem, begin a new career, and discover a passion they never dared to pursue. I've seen some moms dramatically improve their relationships with their husbands, kids, and friends, all because they finally let go of the hurt, pain, and resentment they had harbored within them for years. What's so important to consider also is this: your body doesn't know if the pain happened twenty years ago or five minutes ago. The stress hormones that are released are the same and they don't know the difference. That's why when we talk about letting go and beginning the healing process we're not just talking about a mental or emotional thing. It's physical too.

Once we let go to the hurt, pain, or regret that's kept our bodies in a stressful state, the chronic stress response is turned off. The brain alerts the body that it's no longer in danger and the person is safe. Once this message gets across, stress hormones stop being secreted, which have been causing physical wear and tear on the body. At that point, the body begins to heal.

Do you need to end a relationship? Would letting go of your hurt and pain allow you to begin the healing process? Slowly, steadily, and gently, it's time for a goal.

WEEKLY GOAL

- This week, take a long, hard look at your relationships. See how they make you feel and determine if it's best to make some changes or move on. Also, determine how holding onto that pain, grudge, or resentment is affecting you. I can assure you it's not helping your health, wellness, or growth but only you can decide if cutting the tie to a past hurt is something you're ready for. That painful tie may be your last connection to a particular person and you may be afraid to end the connection by letting go (even if the pain is the only connection you have). You have a lot to think about, act on, and healing ahead of you. But every experience you have makes you stronger, wiser, and better. Trust your gut here. You have all the tools you need. You just may need some extra support to help you through.

We are always in relationships. Whether it's with our immediate or extended family, friends, coworkers, neighbors, community, society, and even nature, we are always in some type of relationship. That's why the way we think, act, and behave in our relationships is so important. It defines who and what we are.

How you decide to conduct your relationships is largely based on the way you feel about yourself. The better you feel about yourself, the better quality relationships you find, attract, and keep. The worse you feel, the less you feel you deserve, and your relationships will provide an example of your self-worth.

Negative relationships are mentally, physically, emotionally, and spiritually destructive while positive relationships enrich, encourage, and reward your body, mind, and spirit. It doesn't matter what brought you to realize that you want more positive relationships as long as you take the steps to discover and nurture them. It also doesn't matter what brought you to realize that you're ready to change some unhealthy, negative relationship qualities that you may have as long as the necessary changes are made.

That's what growth is all about. It's about the continual process of becoming an even better you. You are already so incredible. Your goal is to feel good within your own skin. That occurs when we weed out all the negatives and surround ourselves with the positives. We then feel embraced and enveloped with respect, love, and support. These feelings enable us to feel good, heal, and gain the confidence we need to discover our best selves. These feelings also bring about emotions such as compassion, empathy, and love, which are emotions compatible with wellness and healing. That's when the magic happens because these qualities position you to be your best. It then becomes apparent that there is nothing you can't be, do, or have because you understand that you have all the tools you need within you. You will also discover that the only person who's been holding you back all along has been you.

Spiritual
Fitness Program

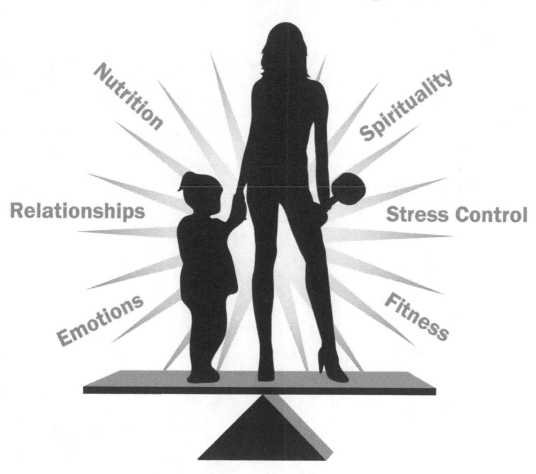

Nutrition

Spirituality

Relationships

Stress Control

Emotions

Fitness

Introduction

What's your definition of spirituality? Is it something you feel when you're in a place of worship, in nature, or with someone you love? Is it a place you can visit, something you can hold, or a feeling that you have? We each have our own definition of spirituality, and there is no right or wrong answer. What seems to be the most general consensus however is that spirituality is the realization that there's more out there than just us. It's the belief that we are each an important piece of a puzzle that can't be completed unless all the pieces are present. It's the feeling that we're all connected in some way, so that if we hurt another, it's as though we're hurting ourselves. It's the belief that, because we're all in this together, we need to help and support one another and the most effective way to do that is through love, appreciation, compassion, and gratitude. It's the feeling that we're all equal, we're not above or below anyone but our goal is to reach our highest place so we have more to give others. It's the quiet peace you feel within when you realize that "you finally get it."

If and when we ever feel this sense of spirituality, we feel blessed. We've found a key to unlock a door that's been there for years, yet we've been unable to open it. We've actually been holding the key all along. Remember that Eagles song "Already Gone?" There's a line, "So often times it happens, that we live our lives in chains and we never even know we have the key." In order to unlock that "spiritual door," we first need to know we have the key. So how do we find it? Throughout the Spiritual Fitness Section, along with greater understanding, development, and awareness, you'll soon find out.

Chapter 1
Let's Start With the Basics

When I became a Whole Health Coach with the National Institute of Whole Health, my professor and mentor Dr. Georgianna Donadio, MSc, DC, Ph.D., (a pioneer in the field of whole health education) opened my eyes to some of the most important concepts I'd ever learned. I was no stranger to education. I've attended college, graduate school, and schools for various certifications, but the concepts she imparted to me changed my entire perspective on life, love, and learning.

One of the most important concepts I learned was how perfectly and precisely the body is interconnected. The body, mind, and spirit are intricately intertwined. The more we understand this, the more we can control our health and wellness, as our illness or healing is largely up to us. So many factors play a part, but I learned that our thoughts control our emotions, which control our behaviors, which control our health, good or bad.

Another concept I learned was how we live according to Abraham Maslow's Hierarchy of Needs. Here's a diagram, then I'll explain.

Abraham Maslow's Hierarchy of Needs

SELF-ACTUALIZATION — personal growth, fulfillment, full potential

SELF-ESTEEM NEEDS — achievement, status, respect, responsibility, reputation

SENSE OF BELONGING — family, affection, friends, relationships

SAFETY AND SECURITY — protection, security, order, law, limits

SURVIVAL — water, food, shelter, air

Although briefly discussed in the Emotional Fitness Program section, here's a more thorough explanation. We're geared for *survival*. The body will do everything in its power to keep you safe. It's a basic need we have and it comes above all else. For example, if you're being attacked, you are not thinking about your bills, or your to-do list. You are thinking about how you will survive.

The next rung on the ladder is the issue of *safety and security*. Once your life is no longer in danger, your next basic need is to feel safe and secure. Some of us never feel safe and secure. If our safety or security is questioned or threatened, we spend our lives trying to fulfill these needs and never make it up the next rung of the ladder.

If our survival is no longer threatened, we feel safe and secure, and we begin our search for a *sense of belonging*. For example, you're not worried about your survival or protection, so you want to feel a sense of belonging with a partner, group, community, society, etc. (By the way, this is why rejection and isolation are so painful, they prevent us from feeling we belong, which is a basic need).

So now we're not being attacked, we have a place to live, food, and some relationships. Many people stop the search right here. They feel they have the basics covered and this is all they need. For those who may have been in toxic, dysfunctional, or detrimental relationships, the damage to their *self-esteem* is one of the motivators that encourage another climb up the ladder. Here's where displays of *self-defense* and *self-protection* come into play (the needs of our egos). We may realize that we've been sacrificing certain needs and search for ways we can feel respected and recognized. Another interpretation is that because we feel safe and secure within our existing relationships, we attempt to improve our self-esteem through goals such as achievement or reputation. These efforts may be seen through the work we do or efforts we display. At some point however, we may realize that we're not defined by our achievements. We begin to understand that self-esteem is an inside job—as opposed to an outside one—and we climb up the next rung.

This leads us to discover our own personal power and self-expression. Many of us never discover our personal power, either because we don't miss it or we don't trust that it's there. Remember when we talked about that "inner guide" from the Emotional Fitness Program Section? It's been guiding you to find that personal power all along. This is called *self-actualization*. You're beginning to realize your value, your worth, and you're on a quest to discover your full potential. You're discovering your inner purpose, your talents, and your creativity. You begin to see through different eyes. You climb the next rung of the ladder.

Through trust, acceptance, and understanding, you realize that we're all interconnected. It doesn't sound so weird or crazy when you hear it anymore. You get it. You understand that we're all here to learn, grow, and evolve although many don't use their time to learn these lessons. You learn that, although we're all so different, we all want to be treated fairly, respectfully, and with value. You apply the "golden rule" because it's so natural and non-threatening to give now. Since you feel safe, secure, peaceful, and content, you have so much compassion, gratitude, and love to give. You lose the "I only take care of my own" mentality because you realize that we're all in this together and "your own" involves everyone you meet. You understand that nothing feels better than to give and you're so much different and better than you've ever been. You're climbing up the *spiritual* ladder now and there's one more rung.

This is the top of the ladder, the pinnacle, the summit. This is where spiritual leaders like Mother Teresa, Gandhi and those with that type of giving spirit reside. They are completely at peace with who they are. They are humble, giving, and compassionate. These people show compassion, love, and respect to all of humanity. There is no distinction between people in their minds because we are all made of the same thing. They respect any and all things because they believe that a giving spirit, life force, greater being, whatever, resides in everything at all times. They are completely spiritual beings and they set a pure and loving example for all of us. So, what rung of the ladder do you want to get to?

WEEKLY GOAL

- Determine where you are currently spending most of your time according to Maslow's Hierarchy of Needs. Are you where you want to? Are you struggling with feeling safe and secure? Do you feel a sense of belonging, or do you feel threatened, insecure, and uneasy? This week, commit to determining where you are according to the Hierarchy of Needs. Once you see where you are, decide what it may take to move up one more rung on the ladder. Stronger relationships? More conviction in your abilities? Decide what it will take because each climb up the ladder brings you closer to your higher purpose, best self, and most exhilarating and fulfilling life.

Chapter 2
Fear: The Greatest Obstacle to Overcome

In order to get "spiritually fit," the first thing that needs to be done is to deal with the many fears you may have. Fear holds us back from the best of everything. Fear can emotionally paralyze us, making us unable to move forward. It may be fear of success, fear of failure, fear of embarrassment, ridicule, rejection, lack, abundance, punishment, independence, dependence, separation, isolation, abandonment, bugs (had to stick that in). The list goes on and on. The point is, our fear is one of our greatest obstacles to overcome. Overcoming a fear can turn obstacles into opportunities. The force of fear (that we've created) can seem monumental if we allow it. But think about this. What happens when we're terrified of something but we do it anyway?

Exhilaration, pride, confidence, and success! The feeling of "yeah, I did it!" That's the feeling you get whenever you overcome any fear. So if that feeling feels so good, why don't we seek it out more often?

It's a case of risk versus reward. In our minds, the potential downside isn't worth the feeling of success on the other side. Here's a question for you. What's the price you pay for giving into your fear, for giving in instead of going for it? For many of us, the price is a lack of happiness, relationships, fulfillment, joy, and purpose. That's a big price to pay in order to stay safe. Now, everyone has different levels of joy, satisfaction, and abundance. For one person, joy can mean an extra hour of sleep, for another it can mean a sunny day, for others it can mean a peaceful day with the kids. There's no problem with any of this unless you feel like you're missing out on something.

Let's start by talking about the fear of failure. Here's where you may want to try something new but the risk of failure holds you back. Why does it hold you back? Maybe you're concerned about facing judgment, ridicule, or "I told you so" from people in your life. These are the naysayers that zap you of your drive, ambition, and motivation if you let them. These people can have a hold on you so firm that you determine that the possible success isn't worth the negativity you'll hear, so you just give up.

While the naysayers have a strong hold on you, the greatest naysayer in the equation just may be you. If you're filled with self-doubt about what you're able to achieve and accomplish, the naysayers just confirm your already borderline belief in yourself. If you were on the fence about trying something or not, the naysayers will easily talk you out of it. You'll then agree and wonder why you ever thought you could try it in the first place.

Your self-doubt is something you've learned and you can unlearn it as well. Just how you bought into your ability that you can't is how easily you can buy into your belief that you can. You have all the tools you need except for a firm belief in yourself. By giving into your fear, you're dismissing your passion. You're telling yourself that your deepest happiness and greatest fulfillment isn't so important. If your child told you about her dreams of greatness, success, and achievement, would you tell her to just forget about it because she wasn't capable? Of course not. But by giving into your fear you're essentially doing that to yourself.

If you were to look at the life of someone who's achieved something wonderful, you'll find that the success didn't necessarily come easy. They may have had many unsuccessful attempts and roadblocks before they found the desired result. What they did have from the beginning however was this equation:

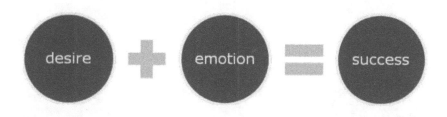

What they also believed was that they didn't fail. Each failed attempt brought them one step closer to finding the correct answer. They didn't personalize the failure; they used it as a stepping stone to achieve their desired result.

Is there something that you've wanted to accomplish but talked yourself out of? Something that may have brought you joy, greater fulfillment, passion, and purpose yet for some reason, it hovers in the back of your mind due to your fear of failure? Come on scaredy-cat, time for a goal.

WEEKLY GOAL

- Think about something you've wanted to do but held back on. I'm sure there are many reasons why, such as the time, the money, etc. However, look deeper and you may find that even greater reasons for not starting was because of the risk, the effort, the ridicule, or judgment you'd face if it didn't work out. When we want something badly enough, we find a way to make it work. By not pursuing a passion or interest, we may blame or resent those we feel have held us back while confirming our own self-doubt. This week, discover what would bring you joy that you haven't begun due to your fear of failure. Then talk yourself out of that and find a way to begin. Sometimes it's best to stop thinking so much and as Nike says: "Just do it."

Chapter 3
Action

S o, let's say you think there's something you may want to try, whether it's going back to school for a degree, a career change, running the marathon, volunteering, or beginning a rewarding hobby. You've figured out what you want to do and you even managed to find a way to overcome your fear of what people will say, think, and feel about your new pursuit. You're still unsure if it will work but you've realized that you don't want to put your needs aside any longer. Doing something "just for you" is what's in order for you to feel fulfilled and satisfied. What do you do now?

For many moms, ideas are great but implementing them is the problem. They have great ideas, know how enriched they'll feel if they venture down this new path but are stuck in how to get things going. Here's where you simply take some practical steps to see things through. For example, let's say you realize that you're the one taking pictures at every party, you get a thrill out of perfectly capturing the moment on film and you want to take your talent to the next level. You love photography and you want to explore it further.

The first thing you need to do is create your action plan. That's the step-by-step practical process for how you'll make this work. Do you have the resources you need such as babysitting for the kids, a free afternoon, and a quality camera? You action plan is like cooking. With cooking, you purchase the ingredients, get them all together, have the right equipment, and follow the steps in order to create your delicious dish. Your action plan is a step-by-step program that enables your idea to go from thought to reality. In fact, when you think of how anything was created, it began as a thought first. Someone saw a need for something (whether it was a personal need or not), took that thought and through a step-by-step process, turned it into a finished product.

Now, getting there may mean overcoming some hurdles, so here's where you need your strong resolve. You may feel like you're "battling the elements" at times, when things aren't going how you planned. The process may be more difficult than you thought it would be as obstacles you hadn't considered may creep up. It doesn't matter. The harder something may be, the sweeter the success when it's finally accomplished. The more challenges you face, the more pride you'll feel when you see what you've managed to overcome. Don't be afraid to push yourself. Getting out of the safe zone can be exhilarating, rewarding, and fun. Also, what's the worst that can happen? The only failure there is occurs when you give up trying. So think of how you'll feel when you finally pursue that dream. Ready? Time for your goal.

WEEKLY GOAL

- So, you know what you want to do and it's time to take action. You need to create your action plan. How will you make this work? Have you covered all your bases? Many moms find it helpful to write it down. Write down your passion at the top of the page and the necessary steps to get there. For every obstacle you find, write it down. Then figure out a way to overcome that obstacle and write it down too. You can also write a time line for yourself, giving you the appropriate time you need to get from step one to step two. This way you "chunk it down" for yourself and it's not as overwhelming. For example: week one, find babysitter. Week two, buy camera. Week three, join photography class. You may even want to write down a certain response you'll say if questioning from others may derail you.

Chapter 4
Discovering Your Purpose

Many moms are at a loss when it comes to understanding what their true purpose is. This often occurs because we live our lives on autopilot. We're so busy just trying to get through our day that we don't have the time, effort, or energy to think beyond. Also, many of us live our lives by being *reactive* as opposed to being *proactive*. Here's where we're dealing with life as it comes at us, as opposed to creating the life we want to live. So, you're looking to become "spiritually fit" and that involves discovering your purpose. Why?

Discovering your true purpose brings us joy, passion, and fulfillment. When we feel enriched, we're happy. When we're happy, our lives are better, we have more to give, we're learning, growing, and evolving. We feel complete, at peace, and relaxed because we're living the life we've dreamed of. We're showing our children how to follow their dreams because we're showing them the great pleasure it's brought us. We feel compelled to contribute and connected to something sacred. We're filled with and fueled by love. Finally, we're living as our highest self. So, how do we discover our purpose so we can have all of these great feelings?

When you think about it, you'll find that there's something you're naturally good at. Something you enjoy, something that makes the time fly, something that no one needs to tell you how to do. It could be a unique strength, gift, or calling. When you do this thing, you feel good. Maybe it's something you always did when you were growing up. For example, let's say you always loved horses. You had posters of horses hanging on your walls, every year you begged for a pony for your birthday. You get the idea? Then you grew up and were told how completely impractical the idea of horses were so you became an accountant instead (no offense to any accountants. I respect you immensely; I can barely add!). My point is, you're love for horses was and still may be there. Now you just need to find a way to incorporate horses in some capacity into your life.

Maybe that means taking horse back riding lessons, going to a horse farm, or reading books about horses. Only you know how to satisfy that need. Now, sometimes the desire is more general like "I want to help people." Very often, through the process of elimination, you can narrow this down to what that means to you. Do you like helping kids, adults, animals? If so, in what capacity, as a doctor, a teacher, a coach, a mentor? It's by following this thinking that leads you to your greater purpose. In fact, that's exactly what has lead you to read what you're reading right now. I'll explain.

I graduated from college with a double major: TV Production and Broadcast Journalism. I loved the idea of writing and producing for television. Working in the field for a while, I had an opportunity to produce a segment for an organization that helped the disabled. I was inspired by the piece and I realized that I wanted to help people, but didn't yet know how. The thought stayed with me; in fact it grew so that I no longer enjoyed producing anything for TV that didn't make a difference.

I always loved health and fitness and I thought I may be able to help people in this capacity, so I began to think of ways to turn it into a career. I fought with myself for weeks saying "I invested all this time learning TV, how can I justify giving it up?" To get my feet wet, I bit the bullet and got a job at NutriSystem. I started helping people lose weight. I wasn't there yet but I was on the right track. My college roommate called one day and said "Deb, want to take a cooking class?"

I said "Sure, sign me up."

She called back and said, "Let's take a class towards something. Let's be Dietitians." I enrolled, and she never left her job.

I then had to find a way to earn money while going back to school. I thought, "What goes well with nutrition that I can do around my schedule, make money at and enjoy?" I became a Personal Trainer. I began to feel like I was on the right track.

Years later, I was working exclusively with moms, inspiring them to look, feel and live their best. But something was missing. Their lifestyles (along with my own) were chaotic and preventing us from living our best. I became a Whole Health Coach. With this in place, every mom I saw began finally thinking, feeling, looking, living and acting the way she'd always wanted to. We all began "getting our mojo back." That's when I became The Mojo Coach® and that's what pushed me to write this book. See what I mean?

Of course there were obstacles, more than I care to remember or discuss. The point is, I felt a gentle pull and heard that "inner guide" steering me along to discover my purpose. It would have been so easy to ignore it because I knew, by listening, my life would never be the same. I made the decision to let it take me by my hand and show me which way to go. I've made about a million mistakes so far but each one brings me closer to getting it right.

There is no doubt that I'm now doing exactly what I've been put here to do. I'm living my dream. By being ready, willing, and open to discovery, you can and will discover your purpose too. When you do, it's nothing short of incredible. It's one of the biggest "*aha* moments" you'll ever have. Here's your goal.

WEEKLY GOAL

- What's your purpose? What do you do that when you're doing it, time seems to fly? What is it that makes your spirit soar? What is it that if it were a career, you'd do it even if you didn't get paid? What is it that brings joy to your heart and peace to your soul? This week, commit to discovering what it is. We all have something. Something that's specific to us. Something we're uniquely qualified for because the desire for it comes easy. Find out what it is. It's why you're here.

Chapter 5
Tragedy or Crisis as a Catalyst to Making Changes

For many of us, our lives don't change unless they have to. We plod along, going about our business and never consider how we're living until we need to make a change. Often those changes become necessary because of a tragedy, crisis, illness or disease.

We often look at a crisis as a terrible disruption in our lives, one that throws us and we wonder if we'll ever recover from it. I'm sure you've heard the saying "as one door closes, another door opens." That door was closed because of a tragedy, trauma, crisis, or disappointment. When you've allowed yourself to heal from the pain, you were able to discover another door. Upon opening the door, it led you to another chapter in your life, one that you wouldn't have stumbled upon if the other door never closed.

What also happens with a tragedy is that it forces us to reevaluate our lives, ourselves, and how we've been living. For example, someone hears a frightening diagnosis. They realize they've neglected certain people, needs, etc. and make the changes to more fully appreciate what they have. Tragedy also forces us to make a decision about how you've been acting. For example, maybe you were holding onto a hurt, grudge or pain. A tragedy can force you to see how pointless that can be and can be the catalyst to bringing about a change in your perspective and behavior.

A crisis can also cause us to reflect on how we've been living. It can make us see that we've been living in a way that doesn't support our values, and encourages us to recognize that it's time for a change.

In some cases, a tragedy can be freeing. You may have felt restricted, stuck, locked into a hopeless and desperate situation. When you had time to heal from the crisis, you may have allowed yourself to see an opportunity that you otherwise would never have allowed.

So often we look at tragedy as something terrible but it is often a blessing in disguise. It's a blessing because it causes us to reevaluate our lives, giving us another opportunity to get it right. Without the tragedy you may not have thought to reconsider how things were going. Only through the pain you felt from the tragedy can you clearly see the hope. From the discomfort you can measure the joy. It can serve as a means of comparison. For example, how can you measure joy if you don't have pain?

The opportunity we get from a tragedy can also force us to live more in the present because we've learned just how precious life is. It makes us not want to miss a thing, because life is short so we take in all the beauty that life can provide. Instead of listening with half an ear when our children speak, we may stop what we're doing and appreciate their message. Instead of fuming in traffic, we may choose to stay present in order to enjoy the music on the stereo.

Tragedy can be a blessing in disguise. There's *always* something positive that comes from it if you allow yourself to find it. If you allow yourself to heal from a tragedy, take a look at the new you. Chances are you'll find a greater knowledge, perspective, and understanding. What you do with that information is up to you, but if it weren't for that tragedy, you wouldn't have that knowledge.

I'm certainly not saying that we aren't supposed to feel the pain tragedy can cause. Without addressing, feeling, and working through that pain, you probably can't heal. What I'm saying is to find the lesson the tragedy brings. Find the opportunity, new knowledge, perspective, or path that the crisis caused you to see. Then take that pain and use it as a stepping stone to greater understanding. Here's your goal.

WEEKLY GOAL

- In every tragedy you face, there's a life lesson. Something that brings you greater awareness and understanding. Think of a tragedy you've experienced and find the lesson you learned, or lesson you were supposed to learn but haven't. It's also a helpful way to deal with the tragedy because by finding the opportunity in it, you're bringing some closure to all that pain. This week, commit to discovering the lesson behind "the rough patches" in your life. Learn and grow from them and allow the information to make you wiser, better, stronger, more loving, giving, and compassionate.

Chapter 6
Gratitude and Abundance

In order to become "spiritually fit," you need to strengthen your sense of gratitude. That's that feeling of recognizing all the gifts you have. It's when you see the abundance and beauty around you. It's when "wanting what you have" weighs more than "having what you want." It's that appreciation you feel for what you may consider "the little things" but are by no means small at all. Things like a sunny day, the beautiful foliage, a warm embrace, a bright smile, a kind gesture, a nice complement, your child's giggle, a hot cup of coffee, the list is endless. How can you experience more gratitude?

It begins with the understanding that you control the emotions you feel. Although you can't control certain situations, by controlling your emotions you are creating your life experiences. The way it works is you're attracting situations to you all the time that reflect how you feel. The life you're living now is an indication of the thoughts you've been feeling in the past. Those thoughts manifested into experiences that led you to where you are right now. Feel gratitude and abundance and you'll attract gratitude and abundance. Feel a sense of lack in joy, love, money, self-worth, and you'll attract feelings and situations that support those thoughts.

So while you may think "but I really want to be…" (happy, loved, thin, or whatever you want), the only reason you may not be those things is because you're focusing on the lack of what you want instead of tasting, feeling, and believing that it can be yours. For example, "I really want to be thin" can be coming from "I really want to be thin because I'm so fat." "I want to be happy" can be coming from "I want to be happy because I'm so miserable." These thoughts, while they may seem positive, are coming from a place of not having something. They're based on the thoughts of *not* being thin and *not* being happy. They're not coming from a place of gratitude and abundance because you feel thin or feel happy. They're coming from the desire to have these things because you feel you don't. That's a sense of lack.

When you think these thoughts, it reaffirms what you don't currently have. The more you reaffirm what you don't have, the more you attract situations that support your current belief. There are no exceptions to this rule. It's the universal law of attraction and it's not some crazy far fetched thing. It's an energy thing. If you're unsure, just take a look at the people around you. Positive, optimistic, happy people with a giving spirit seem to attract those types of people and situations to them. Negative, nasty, pessimistic people seem to always be complaining that "they're never lucky" or "they never get a break." They're only getting back what they're sending out.

When we're not communicating through speaking, we're communicating by body language, along with our senses. You know how you feel an instant chemistry or an instant connection with someone? How about when someone immediately gives you a sense of unease? These people didn't have to say a word; you sensed it. Finally, have you ever "felt" someone behind you or sensed someone staring at you from across the room? It's that same energy that is responding to the thoughts you think. That's why it's crucial to control your thoughts because those thoughts attract whatever it is that matches what you feel.

The sooner you embrace this concept, the sooner you'll see why it's so important to feel good about yourself and about your life. The better you feel about yourself, the more comfortable you are in your own skin. The more comfortable you are, the less you need to keep "the good stuff" for yourself. You have a sense of trust, faith, and abundance within you that drives you to share those feelings with others. You feel a sense of gratitude for all that you have and all that you see. These feelings bring about situations that support how you feel. Positive feelings attract positive experiences, people and situations in your life. Focusing on the negative or lack of what you have brings about more of the same.

So while you may think it's hedonistic or unimportant to simply feel good, it truly is the basis for a more rewarding, enriching, and satisfying life. Every positive thought, emotion, and outcome stems from a foundation of feeling good. It's like planting seeds on the most fertile, moist, and nutrient- rich soil as opposed to dry, hard clay. By feeling good, you're giving yourself the gift of endless possibilities all within your reach. Now all you have to do is want it badly enough that you can breathe, feel, and taste it. That desire fuels the passion to bring to you, whatever it is you want, that much quicker. Now that's a lot to be grateful for!

WEEKLY GOAL

- What are you grateful for? This week, commit to discovering all the beauty and abundance you see. Write it all down and become aware of it all. Take nothing for granted and appreciate all that you have. When you really feel blessed, grateful, and appreciative, watch closely for what happens. All of a sudden, things you may have been struggling with in the past are easily available to you. Love, intimacy, friendships, money, weight loss, health, whatever, it is all within your grasp. There are no mistakes; you are bringing it all about through your positive emotions and sense of gratitude. You are truly in control and you are putting yourself on a path to discover your highest self and most incredible life.

In the Spiritual Fitness Section, you've been asked to do some real soul searching. It can seem as if you've been walking around with blinders on, giving you a limited view of what's available to see. I've asked you to take the blinders off and take it all in. There's so much available to you, so much beauty around to see, to take notice of and to take part in.

I've also asked you to overcome your fears, throw away your limiting beliefs, and disregard your self-doubts. These are huge tasks because they've been a part of you for so long. They feel as natural as any body part you have. You don't think about it, it's just there. But these limiting beliefs have been in the way. They've prevented you from discovering your purpose, being your best self and experiencing what you may find to be your ultimate happiness.

I've asked you to "feel the fear and go for it anyway," because right past that fear is joy and exhilaration. I've asked you to become your best because these things have been within you all along, you've just been too afraid to try.

There is nothing I've asked you to do that you're incapable of. You're already whole, equipped with all the tools you need. You have access to the greatest computer in the world (your mind) and the greatest medicine cabinet available (your thoughts and the chemicals secreted as a result). You can do anything. There is nothing you can't be, do, or have. Anything and everything is within your reach. Your passion and the emotion it's fueled with will determine how long it takes you to reach any goal you have. Nothing is off limits and your actions and behaviors will always determine your results.

This is no dress rehearsal. It's your chance to make life simply okay or spectacular. No one makes these decisions but you. If you've felt like you've given up control for too long, take it back because it's been yours all along. You are capable, powerful, and complete.

I'm here for you and want to share in your success. Feel inspired, empowered, and ready to become the person you'd always hoped you'd be. The only thing that's ever stopped you is you, and now you know better. Now there's no holding back.

Wishing you all the love, life and laughter on this incredible journey to become your best,

Debi The Mojo Coach®

Note: Now that you've completed the book, I want to make sure you keep up the momentum and keep moving forward. Make sure you sign up at www.TheMojoCoach.com for additional ideas, information, resources and inspiration!

The Pay It Forward Program

N othing feels better than to give. When we do, we flood ourselves with "feel good" chemicals which heal and strengthen our bodies, minds and spirits. At the same time we give of ourselves, we brighten someone else's day, making them feel valued, supported and cared for. That's exactly why I created The Lifestyle Fitness, Inc. Charity Program and The Pay It Forward Program. Here's how the Pay It Forward Program works:

If you "got your mojo back" as a result of something you learned from this book then join me in Paying It Forward! Just visit this link: www.TheMojoCoach.com/book_products.php to purchase a copy of this book for another mom and I'll send you a free CD! ($20 value). Once you visit that link, click "I want this book". Then click the green check out box and you'll see a box labeled "Comments/Special Delivery Instructions" below the payment information. Simply write "Pay It Forward Program" in that box. My CD will be shipped to you along with the book you just purchased for another mom who's ready to get her mojo back!

Also, 50% of any profit I would have received from your book purchase goes straight to the Charity Program so through your Pay It Forward Act, I give you a CD, you give another mom a book, we help those less fortunate by contributing to charity…and the cycle continues! How great is that?!

Thanks for being such an important part of this project. Also, thanks for the opportunity to let me into your life. It's been my greatest honor and privilege to work with you. Hopefully now you see in yourself the beauty that's been there all along.

Stay in touch!

Debi

Works Consulted

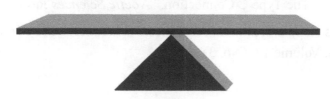

American Journal of Clinical Nutrition: McCarthy et al. (2007).

American Heart Association: Diet and Lifestyle Recommendations. American Psychological Association (2004)

ARA, "Exercise to Combat Stress and Potential Illness."

B.B. (1997). "Social Life Nothing to Sneeze At", Science News. Vol. 152

Bezruchka, S. (2001). "Is Our Society Making You Sick?" Newsweek. 14

Borysenko, L. (1994). *The Power of the Mind to Heal.* California: Hay House, Inc.

Brody, H. (2000). "Tapping the Power of Placebo." *Newsweek*, 66.

Dwyer, W. (1992). *Real Magic.* New York: Harper Collins Publishers

Harding, P. (2002). *Anti Aging and the Adrenal Gland.* Nutrition for Optimum Health
    Association, Inc. "Immune System Health and Low Cortisol."

Holman, D. and Pape, G. (2007). *Repotting, 10 Steps for Redesigning Your Life*. California:
    Hay House, Inc.

International Journal of Pediatric Obesity

Lambert, C. (2007). "The Way We Eat Now." *Harvard Magazine*

Meaney, M. *Stress and Disease: A Seminar for Health Professionals.* "Stress Hormones",
    Institute for CorText Research and Development

Pert, C.B. (1997). *Molecules of Emotion.* New York: Scribner.

——. (2006). *Everything You Need to Know to Feel Go(o)d.* California: Hay House, Inc.

Reed-Stitt, B. (2004). *Food and Behavior, a Natural Connection*. Wisconsin: Natural Press

Temoshok, L. (1993). "The Type C Connection." *Noetic Sciences Review*. 21-26.

Wood, C. (1996). "Is Hope a Treatment for Cancer." *Advances: The Journal of the Mind/Body Health*. Volume 12, (No. 3). 66.

Suggested Reading

The Success Principles: How to Get from Where You Are to Where You Want to Be, by Jack Canfield. New York: Harper Collins (2005).

The Power of the Mind to Heal, by Joan and Miroslav Borysenko, Ph.D. California: Hay House, Inc. (1994).

Molecules of Emotion: The Science Behind Mind-Body Medicine, by Candace Pert, Ph.D. New York: Scribner (1997).

Everything You Need to Know to Feel Go(o)d, by Candace Pert, Ph.D. California: Hay House, Inc. (2006).

Empowering Women: Every Woman's Guide to Successful Living, by Louise Hay. California: Hay House, Inc. (1997).

Repotting: 10 Steps for Redesigning Your Life, by Diana Holman and Ginger Pape. California: Hay House, Inc. (2007).

Why Zebra's Don't Get Ulcers: The Acclaimed Guide to Stress, Stress-Related Diseases and Coping, by Robert Sapolsky. New York: Owl Books (2004).

Mind Over Back Pain: A Radically New Approach to the Diagnosis and Treatment of Back Pain, by John Sarno, MD. New York: Berkley Books (1982).

Healing Back Pain: The Mind-Body Connection, by John Sarno, MD. New York: Warner Books (1991).

The Mindbody Prescription: Healing the Body, Healing the Pain, by John Sarno, MD. New York: Warner Books (1998).

The Cortisol Connection: Why Stress Makes you Fat and Ruins Your Health—And What You Can Do About It, by Shawn Talbott, Ph.D. California: Hunter House, Inc. (2002).

Adrenal Fatigue: The 21st Century Stress Syndrome, by James Wilson, ND, DC, Ph.D. California: Smart Publications (2001).

Ask and It is Given: Learning to Manifest Your Desires, by Esther and Jerry Hicks. California: Hay House, Inc. (2004).

The Law of Attraction, by Esther and Jerry Hicks. California: Hay House, Inc. (2006).

The Pathway: Follow the Road to Health and Happiness, by Laurel Mellin. New York: Harper Collins (2003).

Being in Balance: 9 Principles for Creating Habits to Match Your Desires, by Dr. Wayne Dyer. California: Hay House, Inc. (2006).

How to Expand Love, His Holiness the Dalai Lama. New York: Atria Books (2005).

Mother-Daughter Wisdom: Creating a Legacy of Physical and Emotional Health, by Christiane Northrup, MD. New York: Bantam Dell (2005).

Shrink Yourself: Break Free from Emotional Eating Forever, by Roger Gould, MD. New Jersey: John Wiley and Sons (2007).

The Beck Diet Solution: Train Your Brain to Think Like a Thin Person, by Judith Beck, Ph.D. Alabama: Oxmoorhouse (2007).

You're Wearing THAT?: Understanding Mothers and Daughters in Conversation, by Deborah Tannen. New York: Random House (2006).

Even June Cleaver Would Forget the Juice Box, by Ann Dunnewold, Ph.D. Florida: Health Communications, Inc. (2007).

Briefcase Moms: 10 Proven Practices to Balance Working Mothers' Lives, by Lisa Martin. Canada: Cornerview Press (2004).

Life Is Short—Wear Your Party Pants: Ten Simple Truths That Lead to an Amazing Life, by Loretta LaRoche. California: Hay House, Inc. (2003).

Life Makeovers: 52 Practical & Inspiring Ways to Improve Your Life One Week at a Time, by Cheryl Richardson. New York: Broadway Books (2000).

Your Destiny Switch: Master Your Key Emotions, and Attract the Life of Your Dreams! by Peggy McColl. California: Hay House, Inc. (2007).

About the Author

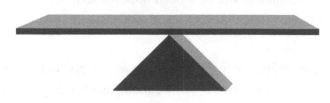

Debi Silber, MS, RD, WHC, is a Registered Dietitian with a Master of Science degree in Nutrition Science. She's a Certified Personal Trainer, Whole Health Coach, and lifestyle expert—just for moms. As the President of Lifestyle Fitness, Inc., Debi has been working exclusively with moms for nearly twenty years, inspiring and empowering them to become fit, healthy, and happy through her Lifestyle Fitness Program. She's been branded The Mojo Coach® because she motivates overweight, overwhelmed, and unfit moms to "get their mojo back" through gradual lifestyle change.

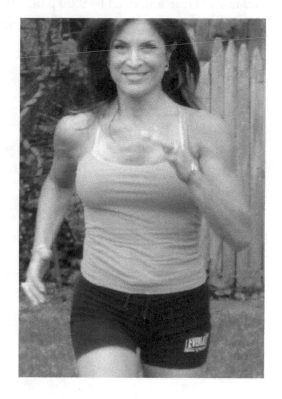

Debi's a featured expert on numerous websites, a popular radio guest, is quoted regularly online and in print, has her own internet TV show and has been featured in a few books about successful "Mompreneurs." She's also on the Advisory Board for the National Institute of Whole Health, The National Association of Home Based Business Moms, is the New York Ambassador for WOMEN.eo and has been honored for her unique charity program.

Debi also holds two certifications in pre/post natal fitness, with specialty recognition in weight loss and weight maintenance. She's been honored as a Madison Who's Who (2007), a Notable American Woman (1992 and 2000) and an Outstanding Young Woman of America (1992 and 1998).

Unmanaged, chronic stress, toxic relationships and a bad case of trying to be "super mom" caused physical, mental and emotional wear and tear leaving Debi with illness, pain… and disease. She's gone from illness to health, pain to pain free living, misery to joy and she's eager to show you how you can do it too through her highly effective, six step approach to health, wellness and happiness…just for moms.

Debi's infectious zest for life, coupled with her ability to blend motherhood with womanhood, has lead her to become widely respected and admired by thousands of moms. Debi also remains fully committed to her own family. She lives in New York with her husband Adam, as well as her four children and four dogs. Besides a day when she can get her children, dogs and house clean and quiet by 9:00 p.m., she considers her strong marriage and highly spirited children to be her greatest accomplishment.

BONUS!!!

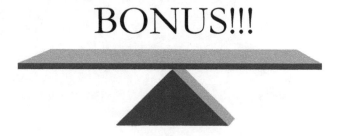

YOUR FREE AUDIO DOWNLOAD

Here's your golden ticket to hear answers to some of the greatest obstacles moms face today regarding nutrition, fitness, and wellness.

Enjoy your free audio download by visiting www.lifestylefitnessbook.com to begin the first step on your journey towards discovering your best self.

I'm thrilled and honored to be working with you!

Wishing you all the best,

Debi

The Mojo Coach®